JIHAD AND AMERICAN MEDICINE

JIHAD AND AMERICAN MEDICINE

Thinking Like a Terrorist to Anticipate Attacks via Our Health System

ADAM FREDERIC DORIN, M.D.

The Praeger Series on Contemporary Health and Living
Julie Silver, M.D., Series Editor

Praeger Security International
Westport, Connecticut • London

Library of Congress Cataloging-in-Publication Data

Dorin, Adam Frederic, 1963–

Jihad and American medicine: thinking like a terrorist to anticipate attacks via our health system / Adam Frederic Dorin.

p. ; cm. – (Praeger series on contemporary health and living, ISSN 1932–8079)

Includes bibliographical references and index

ISBN-13: 978–0–275–99637–6 (alk. paper)

1. Terrorism–Health aspects–United States. 2. Medical errors–United States–Prevention. 3. Medical care–United States–Quality control. 4. Health facilities–Safety measures–United States. 5. Health care reform–United States.

[DNLM: 1. Terrorism–prevention & control–Popular Works. 2. Health Care Reform–Popular Works. 3. Medical Errors–prevention & control–Popular Works. 4. Safety–Popular Works. 5. Security Measures–Popular Works. WA 295 D697j 2007]

I. Title. II. Series.

RC88.9.T47D67 2008

363.325–dc22   2007028386

British Library Cataloguing in Publication Data is available.

Library of Congress Catalog Card Number: 2007028386

ISBN-13: 978–0–275–99637–6

ISSN: 1932–8079

First published in 2008

Praeger Security International, 88 Post Road West, Westport, CT 06881

An imprint of Greenwood Publishing Group, Inc.

www.praeger.com

Printed in the United States of America

The paper used in this book complies with the Permanent Paper Standard issued by the National Information Standards Organization (Z39.48–1984).

10 9 8 7 6 5 4 3 2 1

This book is for general information only. No book can ever substitute for the judgment of a medical professional. If you have worries or concerns, contact your doctor.

The names and many details of individuals discussed in this book have been changed to protect the patients' identities. Some of the stories are composites of patient interactions created for illustrative purposes.

This book is dedicated to the families of those who have lost loved ones to terrorism—domestic and foreign. It is a reflection of the spirit and love of my parents, Doris and Hal; it is a symbol of devotion to my wife, Shirin, and my beautiful children Phillip, Alexander, and Emily. May my family and yours live on to see the day where hatred and murder wilt in the light of our one God.

I also dedicate this work to the concept of vigilance, without which there will never be peace and security on this Earth. I recall the words of my father growing up: "We rarely regret the things we do, but we invariably regret the things we do not do."

CONTENTS

Acknowledgments

This book project has been a labor of love. I am grateful for the opportunity to contribute to the growing body of knowledge addressing how best to protect our nation from future terrorist infiltration and attacks. The research I conducted in the areas of health care systems, medicine, security, global terrorism, and world history was extensive. None of it would have been possible without the patience and cooperation of my beautiful wife, Shirin A. Dorin, D.D.S. She is a keen intellect and has an astute sense of writing style. Her assistance, especially with the appendix section on the "history of medical terrorism from the beginning of time," was invaluable.

I'd like to recognize my children, Phillip Daniel, Alexander Michael, and Emily for their support and suggestions. They are the light of my life.

My parents, Harold P. Dorin and Doris E. Dorin, are the two greatest people I know. They put in many hours reviewing my work and making excellent critiques and edits. I cannot thank them enough for everything. I'd also like to recognize my sister, Joanna D. Brandt, M.D. and my brother, Paul E. Dorin, Esq for their reviews, encouragement, and suggestions during this endeavor.

My cousin Cimarron Buser offered good suggestions that I took to heart. My friend from college, Glenn Davison, M.D., was a source of encouragement and a tremendous boon to this project by introducing me to Mr. John Marke, health care, government, and business consultant with Deloitte-Touch, LLP.

My cousin Mitch Feig was a unique source of interesting articles on terrorism and the global, Islamic jihadist movement; my friends Khatera and Mehdi Miramadi have been there for my wife and I throughout this project—thank you! To all the doctors, nurses, and technicians at the SHARP Grossmont Plaza Surgery Center, thank you for putting up with all my ranting about this project; and to Jason, a very smart surgical technician, thank you for your insightful ideas and comments. A "thank you" also goes out to Marcy Mishiwiec and Rebecca Haines, M.D. for their excellent referrals to experts in various aspects of health systems security, information technology, and public policy.

A special thanks goes out to our friends Boris and Edit Zelkind, Christine and Michael Lindmark, and Bill and Diane Holmes. I don't know where my wife and I would be without the weekends—and friends to spend them with. In their own unique ways, these members of our West Coast extended "family" have offered intellectual "gifts," which have made their way into this small tome. I am also genuinely blessed to have reconnected with real family members Christine and Tom Lucas, Jennifer Lucas, and Elyse Boozer, who now live close by.

Robert Kotler, M.D. ("Doctor 90210") deserves mention for digging into his archive of materials on book marketing. His personal experiences and willingness to "brainstorm" on how best to get this important information to the general public is noted and very much appreciated.

Lastly, I'd like to recognize Greenwood Publisher's editor, Debbie Carvalko and her staff for their ongoing assistance, support, and guidance. Thank you, Debbie, for giving me this opportunity to make a contribution to terrorism prevention.

INTRODUCTION: AMERICAN HEALTH CARE FACILITIES MAY BE THE NEXT GROUND ZERO

Have you ever asked yourself how you would like to die?

If so, it is doubtful the answer was "... as a result of an act of terrorism!"

Even more unlikely is the possibility that you would envision dying unexpectedly at your doctor's office, surgery center, or local hospital. Health care facilities are one of the few safe havens—one of the few places of refuge—left in our hectic, crazy world... or so we would like to think. This book will explore the known data on the subject of health care safety and security. It will also carve out new territory in the name of *prevention* on a national security landscape that is now dominated by a "post-attack" mentality regarding health care emergency services. The reader may find it shocking to discover how little we know about the hundreds of thousands of annual deaths attributed to "medical error" in this country. How many medical errors are really medical murders? Is the risk of medical "terrorism" only from foreign enemies, or has it been operating silently in our health care system under the guise of the ubiquitous death certificate phrase "unknown reaction" or "cardio-pulmonary collapse"?

I am a private practice physician, administrator, and health care manager. I am also a former military officer, and a writer about such diverse fields as anesthesiology, modern surgery, disaster preparedness, critical care medicine, and public policy. This book will pull together all of these disciplines in a way that will enlighten (and may shock) the reader. These pages will bring to light a world most have almost certainly never encountered, or even imagined. The writing here is not geared toward those with a doctorate in the medical sciences, and will *not* be heavy in thesis-paper type discussions of how to treat this or that disease. On the contrary, the reader should find my style to be sapient, if not succinct; I will spare nothing in bringing to the forefront very real and grave dangers the United States—and Western, developed countries in general—face at the hands of Islamofascist terrorists (or killers of any other ilk, domestic or foreign).

By their very definition, terrorists are people and organizations bent on instilling unconscionable fear and destruction in innocent strangers; these are people who will stop at nothing to hurt Americans. These killers represent a very dark path in the ongoing history of mankind. By definition, health care facilities are places where helpless and unsuspecting human beings gather to receive healing care. The hospital is probably the most identifiable symbol of health care and embodies a path of hope, redemption, and love. It is by the very grace of God that these two paths, these lines in the shifting sands of human endeavor, have not yet openly crossed in a way that screams "terror" and evokes public panic. Sadly, this intersection is only a matter of time.

This book will not be laden with multiple citations or complex statistics, although the facts will be solid and well supported by references. Instead, these chapters will paint a picture of real-life vulnerabilities that exist within the fabric of health care in today's America. Through observation, data, and intuition, conclusions will be drawn about basic security weaknesses inherent in American medicine.

Make no mistake: "bioterrorist training" and "rapid response teams" will not protect us against the next terrorist attack. At best, these measures are merely window dressing to placate nervous academicians and legislators. The public knows this.

There can be no solace in the thought that some doctors and nurses have organized to form a "response network" to cooperate in the aftermath of the next terrorist attack.

Instead, we must close every loophole in our system of defense. We must know that we have done everything in our power to minimize the possibility of attack against medical targets and patients. The solution is to preclude (or minimize) the possibility of a major, coordinated terrorist threat.

In a sense, we need to *reengineer* the way hospitals and other health care facilities operate in this country. We need to decide how best we can secure potentially lethal assets within these facilities (e.g., drugs), and how we can minimize the possibility of tampering with existing equipment. We need to secure the multiple perimeters ("circles of safety," if you will) that surround sensitive locations, and think defensively and in military terms. We need to evaluate how well our security guards, cameras, and other monitoring equipment are serving our needs to insure a safe environment for patients, visitors, and staff. We need to ask important questions: From which source do our medications come? Where are they produced? How sure are we of their purity? How well are medications tracked from the factory to the bedside? These and other important questions will be assessed. Planning, preparation, and prevention are our *only* answer.

In this book, you will also read about things that may be called the "dark secrets" of modern medicine. These are observations I have made over the years—things that most people will have never read about and will likely have not ever thought existed within the walls of their local health care institution. These "secrets" may at first blush seem incongruous to the main theme of "terrorism and American medicine," but, as it will be demonstrated, nothing could be further from the truth. One of the themes in this book will be that immorality, corruption, malice, and incompetence on the part of American health care workers and managers, all conspire to lay the groundwork for the ultimate horror of a terrorist attack. I will offer personal anecdotes and describe things I have seen others do. The politics of medical care in this country is very "protective of its own"—this book will let some sunlight into the closed box of American health care in the hope that consumers and policy makers may make better decisions as to how we can best move forward.

Americans should not have to wait two years after a major, preventable health care disaster to read a report of "distinguished experts and political appointees" and only then find out what we should have known from the beginning. In reading these pages, keep an eye out for the insider information, "hot spots," and "trouble zones" of the modern health care establishment as they are revealed—you may be surprised at how many of them you discover!

Jihad and American Medicine starts out with an introduction to the concept of what I call "Medi-Terror"—i.e., terror against medical targets and patients. Terrorists achieve their goal of inflicting psychological damage by taking away our sense of wellbeing and comfort. To create pandemonium and fear, remember that it is not necessary for terrorists to inflict huge numbers of casualties. The Washington, D.C., area snipers of 2002 proved this point, nearly paralyzing that region of the country for weeks. The snipers' random, lethal attacks left less than two dozen individuals killed or injured. If you lived there at that time, however—as I did—it certainly felt like war.

My sister-in-law was possibly the first true victim of the Washington, D.C., "Beltway Snipers." Nearly two weeks prior to the first fatal shooting, she drove over to our house and had me look at a funny-shaped hole that had apparently been inflicted on the driver's-side door panel of her Mercedes SUV. She was concerned because she had heard a loud bang while driving and thought that a large rock had hit her car. The police later discovered that the hole had been made by a bullet. If it were not for the reinforced side beams on that vehicle, she may have never lived to discover—months later—that she had been an early victim of an unsuccessful attempt at murder. (In October 2002, Lee Boyd Malvo and John Muhammad were caught while sleeping in their Chevrolet Caprice at a Maryland rest stop about sixty miles north of Washington, D.C. They were arrested and charged with carrying unlicensed weapons. Among their possessions, a 223-caliber rifle, ammunition, and a shooting tripod were found. Law enforcement forensic tests later linked their rifle to eleven of the fourteen bullets recovered from the scenes of recent attacks. The two were brought to court in Maryland and Virginia; in early 2004, a jury gave Malvo life imprisonment and Muhammad was given the death sentence.)

My sister-in-law's story never made the headlines, but her experience lives on as an eerily subtle reminder of risk (and potential insight) that runs through all of our daily lives. Sometimes identifying a risk is as simple as making a connection that others cannot (or choose not to) make. Someone in the police department in our neighborhood of Potomac, Maryland could have made a connection or deciphered a clue that would have led to the identification of the Beltway Snipers much earlier. Someone could have tied previous attacks together, such as the one involving my sister-in-law, but they didn't. Fighting medi-terror must involve identifying risks and threats (as well as studying previous attacks on health care targets and patients), and extrapolating this insight to the increasing risk of terrorism.

This book will also tackle other issues of grave importance to the American health care system. We will look at how your doctor can, literally, kill you—without even knowing he's doing it! Specifically, we will examine the area of counterfeit drugs, "spiked" medicines, poisoned intravenous fluids, and other potentially lethal agents that are intrinsic to medical facilities. It is likely that the assassins or homegrown terrorists who will be involved in the next attack on the American homeland are already here on U.S. soil. These individuals will have access to medicines and supplies that are unfortunately all too accessible to diversion and misuse.

I will also comment on my experience in an East Coast, inner-city hospital on 9/11. It was there, on that fateful day, that witnesses reported a group of Middle Eastern doctors gathered around a doctors' lounge television and cheered as the planes were shown to hit their targets (none of these doctors were board-certified; all of them were here on work visas by the good graces of the American government). Disturbing? Unbelievable? Yes, but true.

This book will look at hospital/surgery center security (or lack thereof), the various regulatory agencies purportedly created to insure safety in our medical institutions, and the security risks of the average doctor's office. The book will end with a wrap-up of what must be done Stat (Immediately!) to fix the state of affairs of American medicine today, and what every health care consumer and doctor can do to make a difference in preventing terrorism from ever reaching our medical institutions. An appendix will include a short piece on Drug-ATMs as well as a table of terrorist and terrorist-like acts that have been committed against patients since the beginning of time.

Lastly, I'd like to make a final comment to anyone reading this short tome who may be inclined to think that there is information enclosed herein that in any way gives away heretofore unknown or protected information to our enemies. This is a ridiculous idea, but one, which I mention to make a few points perfectly clear. This subject matter of this book is about health care as it is practiced in a free and open society. I am not exploring national secrets as they pertain to nuclear physics, or the blueprints to construct a bomb. All topics and discussions in this text are based on vulnerabilities within our system of medical care that are obvious to anyone who would care to see them. All examples of crimes and acts of terror that have occurred to medical patients or within the walls of medical facilities are taken from the pages of magazines and newspapers over the past few decades—all public knowledge. Anyone who would care to make the inferences I have made—and who took the time to connect the dots as I have done—will come to the same conclusions.

One of the most dangerous attitudes I have witnessed in American history regarding threats to our people and our national security is the belief that acting like a risk doesn't exist makes it so. There have been and will be evil-minded people in this world who want to do us harm; as many of my examples demonstrate, many of them are living and working alongside us every day. We may not be able to identify, track, and stop the efforts of every criminal or terrorist before they choose to act, but we can shore up those weaknesses in our national defense as they apply to American medical system and the delivery of health services to our citizens.

It is my intent to strengthen the fabric of our society by getting inside the head of those who would seek to commit the next attack against Americans. Health care lies at the very core of our communities and our lives. Let us, as a nation, understand and preserve it, as we move through the troubled waters ahead.

NOTE TO THE READER REGARDING REFERENCES AND NOTES

The reader will find this book extremely easy to follow, and also well referenced.

To avoid multiple, cumbersome, and distracting in-text numeration and annotation, sources will be credited in the following manner: References will be cited in the passages themselves (and, where most appropriate, flagged with superscripts); endnotes, where applicable, will be developed by chapter at the end of the book. Some chapters will have few endnotes; others will have many. Because of the unique and "new'" nature of most of the material presented in this text, repeating the same superscripts (for overlapping information) will be minimized—this would be misleading at best and possibly confusing. *Jihad and American Medicine* is not a scientific paper. The world may be a better place if this subject matter was better developed by academicians, and this work was merely an extensive thesis paper. Sadly, this is not the case. Hopefully, this book—and its novel concepts—will set the stage for improved medical safety mechanisms that will benefit all Americans on the larger "system" level of American health care.

As this book goes to print, the recent worldwide focus on terrorists who are health care workers (doctors and lab workers practicing in the United Kingdom and Australia) only serves to reinforce the themes set forth in this book.

1

MEDI-TERROR: THE STAGE IS SET

He that will not apply new remedies must expect new evils, for time is the greatest innovator.

— Sir Francis Bacon

... We saw the patient go out of her room and meet up with someone down the hall. I supposed it was her boyfriend. We were rounding on all of our patients on that floor, and so we decided to come back a few minutes later. When the group of us returned, she was passed out on the floor with a needle in her neck. Her chart said she was a drug addict, but how did she get a hold of drugs? Where was the guy, and how did he get the stuff to her room? Later, after she was revived and on her way to the intensive care unit, we realized that the syringe and needle (and maybe the drugs?) were ours. How did that happen?

— Medical student

No discussion on American health care as the next "ground zero" would be appropriate without first setting the stage of our present predicament. Our enemies, foreign and domestic, have the ability to capitalize on the vulnerabilities of U.S. hospitals and other medical institutions by exploiting our weaknesses. And, as things stand right now, we have many, many weaknesses.

Years ago, an author by the name of Samuel Shem published a novel entitled *The House of God: The Classic Novel of Life and Death in an American Hospital* (copyright 1978, Dell Publishing). Although entertaining, and in some ways bawdy, this novel captured a realistic—and often hilarious—window into the world of "modern medicine" at that time. What made this work an instant favorite (and a modern classic to this day) is that it portrayed a world, however glamorized, that was real. What doctors and nurses said, did, and lived through during their arduous years of training, as portrayed by the fictional characters in that book, were accurate. However artful the author was in painting an appealing story, it would have fallen short if it had not been for its veracity, its telling nature.

The following "hypothetical" scenario is neither contrived nor fictional. Neither is it the literal example of one hospital or surgery center for obvious litigious-fearing reasons. With names that have been changed, what you are going to read is 100 percent factual and real, based on numerous confidential interviews and personal anecdotes. Times have changed since Shem's debut in the late seventies. His "world" faced astronomic interest rates and the dawn of the Iranian hostage crisis (foreshadowing perhaps). At the time the *House of God* first made its way onto bookshelves, the concept of Islamic radicals and terrorists seeking to carry out murder on the American homeland was completely absent from the psyche of our nation.

Hospital Land, USA

Bobby was an emergency room physician, who donated one Saturday morning every other week to give free health care services to a town of poor, migrant workers who lived just south of the Arizona border. He was a hardworking, good man; he valued the immigrant heritage of his family and vowed to always give something back to those less fortunate. Because the charity group that coordinated his medical missions was frequently short on supplies, he occasionally took those medicines he needed from the cabinets and shelves of the hospital emergency department where he was employed. Sometimes, when the operating room was quiet in the dead of night, he would stop by there on his way to the cafeteria vending machines. The operating room was another prime location to take a few vials of drugs without drawing too much attention to himself. He justified the stealing because it was for a good cause.

Oftentimes, Bobby would think to himself how frighteningly easy it was to take medicines that were potentially lethal if fallen into the wrong hands. For example, a twenty-cent vial of succinylcholine (a common muscle relaxant used to place breathing tubes between the vocal cords of patients in the operating room, or used in the emergency room to secure the airway of trauma victims) was conveniently located in various, well-known medicine carts and refrigerators. Although medical facilities are required to safeguard most medicines under lock and key (per various voluntary and government-mandated accreditation requirements), the reality is that drugs are easy to "score." For example, other than at times when official inspectors were on the premises, Bobby found that most cabinets were left unlocked because the logistics of caring for patients and constantly locking and unlocking cabinets was impractical. Furthermore, it could be potentially unsafe to have a STAT code called for a dying patient and be unable to locate a particular key to unlock a draw of life-saving medicines. For this reason alone, medicines were easily accessible (and keys widely known for their location) to anyone who worked for even a short period of time in a hospital, surgery center, emergency room, or medical clinic. Private doctors' offices and procedure rooms were similarly, if not more, lax in their drug-safeguarding measures.

During daylight hours, Bobby could easily take more medicines than needed for the care of a given patient, and thus manage to "squirrel" away extra for his charity work. There was virtually no auditing of nonnarcotic medicines, even those known to be dangerous if used incorrectly. Even for narcotics, since drug levels were not tested (even randomly) in patients, he could sign in to the electronic Pyxis system (drug dispensing machine) for a given patient, but never actually administer the drug he had signed out. Similarly, Bobby could simply give less drug than was stated on the patient chart. During evening hours, Bobby's medical badge got him into sensitive areas and drew no undue attention from security guard cameras.

As for those "cameras," Bobby knew how superfluous they were in most circumstances. As a friend of a hospital security officer, he discovered that (with the exception of the maternity suite) most of the hospital ceiling cameras—despite their blinking red lights—were only for show. As his friend once revealed, "it would be just too expensive for us to monitor, store, and review all those hours of tape for every niche and floor in this place." Furthermore, his friend added, there were legal constraints on patient and staff privacy that precluded widespread surveillance. "Do you know the HIPPA Act?" he once said. "That's the Health Insurance Privacy and Portability Act." "It doesn't say we can't use surveillance for security purposes," he went on, "but have you ever wondered why there are no cameras in operating rooms, where lots of supplies and drugs are stored by nursing and anesthesia at all times. That's because of concerns of lawsuits by patients over an invasion of privacy. If these tapes ever got into the wrong hands, the hospital might as well just write a huge check and not even waste the time defending itself."

For these reasons, Bobby knew where to find the medicines and supplies he needed to help the poor people he so deeply cared for. The only problem was that Bobby's life was not so simple.

Bobby's girlfriend was an extremely intelligent computer technician, who later became a registered nurse and gained employment at a nearby surgery center. Alena had a troubled past, having grown up with a manipulative mother who found her way into the arms of men other than her stepfather; her mother had also been convicted of theft from the convenience store where she once worked. Alena, too, was prone to getting involved with the wrong people, occasionally cheating on Bobby with men she met at her sister's bowling alley. Alena justified her behavior on an "on-again, off-again" drug habit, and on the suspicion that she had been molested by her stepfather as a young girl. Amongst other problems, Alena just couldn't remember much about her younger years. For whatever reason, she suffered from a profound amnesia of events that predated her fifteenth birthday. At the age of eighteen, Alena had been married to a fine young man, but he had run off after six months—only later to have been found dead, a presumed suicide. At the age of twenty-seven, Alena was now unknowingly on the cusp of abetting a criminal act far beyond anything she could have imagined.

One of Alena's male friends turned out to be a drug representative for an international manufacturer of orthopedic and neurosurgical equipment. He, too, had a drug habit; the two of them fantasized that one day, maybe, they could escape to a Caribbean island with enough money to sip margaritas on the sand day after day. Chip was a good "rep," as they were known in the operating room, and his business territory extended to just about every location where surgery was performed in the city. His commissions were tied directly to sales, and he was an aggressive competitor. Thanks to the good intentions of Bobby, Alena and Chip could count on a constant supply of medical supplies that were reliably replenished in the box marked "Mexico" in the corner of the townhouse den which Alena and Bobby shared. Chip had asked Alena if he could occasionally tap into Bobby's supply for an ailing uncle who suffered from cancer. Alena complied. And, hence, a scheme of terror was beginning to take shape.

Chip, otherwise known in his homeland as Ahmed Raymean, was a frustrated, foreign-trained physician who could not pass the board exams to become qualified to practice internal medicine in the United States. Unbeknownst to Alena, Chip was plotting to carry out an attack against the "greedy Americans" who had spoiled the country of his birth. His nearly unfettered access to sensitive hospital locations would allow him to secretly replace bags of intravenous (IV) fluids injected with largely undetectable muscle relaxants. He knew that a very small needle could penetrate the soft plastic wrap that enclosed the unused IV bag and no one would ever know the colorless contaminate had been added. If, as he hoped, he was successful in creating respiratory failure and/or death in patients recovering in their hospital beds, he was confident that any levels of his "poison" would be overlooked as many of these patients would be given this very drug as a part of the resuscitation process. Furthermore, if the patients were immediately "post-op," their bodies would be expected to show traces of this medicine from their recent anesthetic. Chip knew that the technology of radio-frequency identification chips (RFID) had not been widely adopted in medical settings, and hence there would be no way of detecting the removal of Bobby's medicine vials and IV fluids, nor the replacement of "spiked" drugs back into the hospital setting. Because of regulations that required medical waste to be quickly sequestered and disposed of, Chip also knew that the need to keep his fingerprints from getting on the supply material was unnecessary.

Chip's plan was to mastermind a singular day of mayhem and murder—a day when his poisoned IV bags would be left in the operating room supplies of five different surgery centers citywide. In a trial run, Chip had already caused the untimely death of a thirty-six-year-old man in the recovery room of Alena's surgical center. As Alena dutifully recounted to him during one of their regular evening "escapes" to the local bar, the patient was in the bathroom (with his IV still in place) and getting ready to be discharged home. Somehow, she recalled, he had fallen and hit his head. He was not breathing and they tried to revive him, but to no avail. Chip's practice run had worked, and now he would prepare for his large-scale assault. He would plant his lethal weapons, wait to hear about the simultaneous deaths in multiple health care facilities across town, and then call the local newspaper from a public phone claiming responsibility for the acts of deliberate terrorism against American targets.

Had he been successful, Chip's plan would have been a jolt of horror felt by innocent Americans and health care consumers across the globe. As a strange twist of luck, Chip was never allowed the opportunity to unleash his plot in that city on that day. Bobby had happened to be home early one day and discovered Alena and Chip together. Because of Chip's accusations against Bobby about his home supply of medical contraband, and because all parties eventually lost touch with one another, the litany of wrongdoings involving Bobby, Alena, and Chip faded into oblivion; no one mentioned the stolen medicines to authorities. As it turned out, however, Alena had actually been aware of what Chip was plotting (at least to some extent) because she found him one night injecting medicine into an IV fluid bag. This is known because Alena later disclosed this information to a closed meeting of administrators. Out of fear of bad publicity, and chalking it up to just "one bad apple," none of this information ever made its way to the proper authorities. No one ever processed the complete set of information (Alena did not "give up" the role that Bobby had played), so an assessment of a system-wide gap of security in that institution—or in medical institutions nationwide—was never made.

How many variations of Hospital Land, USA (of similar doctors, nurses, and other "paramedical" personnel), exist in health care institutions across America today? How many of them have personal and deep-seated psychiatric problems that obscure what would otherwise be good judgment? To what extent, if any, are health care workers screened and monitored in an ongoing fashion for a susceptibility to borderline psychotic, antisocial, or otherwise unsafe behavior? Should not the employment of hospital workers—entrusted with the care of the weak and most vulnerable, and capable of great wrongdoing—be more strictly regulated in the United States of America? Should not health care institutions be better secured against medicinal tampering and other types of "attack"?

Lest we think of health care crimes as being relegated to the rare, crazy nurse or doctor, we should refer to recent world history to suggest otherwise. The field of health care is far from "off limits" to terror groups, as these organizations have shown no proclivity to respecting the sanctity of other helpless populations. In 2002, when Al Qaeda cells were disrupted in the aftermath of attacks in Bali, it was discovered that attacks were planned against American children attending schools abroad. On more than one occasion, American forces in Iraq have obtained evidence of insurgents planning attacks against targets on the U.S. mainland. In Iraq in 2004, the computer files of a Muslim extremist were recovered, containing detailed maps of elementary and secondary level public schools in several American states.[1] The September 1, 2004, Chechen rebel (also Islamic extremists) attack against a Beslan school in Russia resulted in the death of almost two hundred children.[2] The list of examples could go on and on. There are no safe havens. There are no sanctuaries remaining where we can seek refuge. Terrorists are cowards and bullies, whose favorite targets are often the least well-defended.

Chance, Careless, or Criminal?

Medical "errors" are the eighth leading cause of death for Americans. In hospitals alone (not including clinics, surgery centers, doctors' offices, or nursing homes), unknown or potentially preventable deaths in the American health care system each year surpass those from car accidents (approximately 43,000), breast cancer (approximately 42,000), or AIDS (approximately 16,000).[3]

2

HOW YOUR DOCTOR CAN KILL YOU (WITHOUT EVEN KNOWING WHAT HE'S DONE)

Before an affliction is digested, consolation ever comes too soon; and after it is digested, it comes too late; but there is a mark between these two, as fine almost as a hair, for a comforter to take aim at.

—Laurence Sterne, Irish satirist and author

O mischief, thou art swift To enter in the thoughts of desperate men!

—William Shakespeare (*Romeo and Juliet*)

. . . My "roommate" had just had his intestines operated on—tumor or something. He was in terrible pain all night, moaning and groaning. The nurses and doctors kept coming in and waking me up. Once around two in the morning, I felt a tugging on my IV and I turned around to see some guy in a white coat starting to put a needle in my line. I yelled "stop you idiot, you've got the wrong guy!" There was a long pause and then the words "sorry, the IV poles were right next to each other." I was thinking "man, is it that easy to make a mistake? The guy could have hurt me!"

— patient

This chapter will look at those tools available to terrorists to inflict harm to victims in a health care setting. We are not interested in the obvious (that is, a bomb), but rather those materials already present in hospitals, surgery centers, and doctors' offices that can be used—likely without the knowledge of the medical provider—against helpless patient victims. The idea is that if something *can* be done, it likely will be; our job is to identify those avenues for terror so that we can make them impassable. Later chapters will examine "real life examples" of how innocents have been victimized at the hands of doctors, nurses, and other medical personnel, and how medical facilities themselves are inadequately secured.

THE SIMPLE INTRAVENOUS FLUID BAG

Every surgical patient, and virtually every patient who is admitted to a hospital, has an intravenous line (otherwise commonly referred to as an "IV"). The IV serves the purpose of affording a continuous port of access through which antibiotics, anesthetics, antinausea agents, heart medications, etcetera. can be administered. With an IV line, patients do not have to be "re-stuck" every time medicine is given. In addition, IVs allow doctors and nurses to give medicines and fluids (in treating dehydration, or in patients who have limited or no fluid intake by mouth) over the course of hours or even days.

The very nature of an IV line, however, creates an opportunity for mischief as one can imagine harmful agents could be administered surreptitiously. As with most topics in this book, this is but one example of something seemingly innocent, which few of us would ever contemplate as possibly happening. After all, how could we consider something so firmly associated in our psyche with acts of goodness (and thoughts of "healing," "getting well," and "medical treatment") with an act of malice and violence?

The problem with IV-type fluid bags (and there are so many varieties—those that go into veins, those that feed into joints to provide a clear, visible medium for arthroscopic surgeries, those that irrigate the bladder after prostate surgery, etcetera.) is that they all come from the factory individually packaged in a fine, plastic cover. The IV bag itself is made of a firmer plastic and has two "lips," or portals, at the lower end. One lip is designed to be punctured by IV tubing that leads the fluid (usually some variation of "saline" or salt water) toward its target destination in the body; the other lip is covered with a rubber stopper and can be penetrated repeatedly for the purpose of drawing off—or adding—medicines to the IV bag. If even a small needle were to penetrate the firm bag material itself, it would create a leak. This leak would be easily detected and the bag would be discarded or replaced in short order. On the other hand, the rubber stopper can be used to inject drugs once the bag is placed into use, or even while it is still covered with the thin veil of factory plastic. Unless an IV bag cover was immediately identified as having been tampered with, and thus scurried off to a lab for examination for further visualization and inspection, it would be impossible to detect a small needle used to pierce both the coating and the rubber stopper. Once a bag cover is discarded in the trash, it is just another piece of rubbish surrounded by other medical waste material.

In subsequent chapters, we will see the tragic, real-life consequences of medicines given via IV lines by health care workers in attempts (unfortunately, all too successfully) to kill them. We all read so many horror stories in the newspaper that it may be difficult for us to place them all into perspective. Most readers probably don't know that dozens of people have been killed in the United States by the purposeful injection of lethal drugs into seemingly innocuous IV fluid lines. For now, let's just examine some of the common, inexpensive, and easily accessible medicines located within every health care facility in the United States today. Let's also keep in mind the criminal "advantage" of adding medicines to a bag of IV fluids when no one else is around, then letting the medicine be administered (often times slowly) at a later time when the perpetrator is no longer present at the crime scene. Law enforcement officers sometimes speak of certain types of criminals who *want* to be present to observe the results of their mischief (for example, in the case of arson, police will videotape the gathering crowds in the hope that the wrong-doer is actually amongst them and can later be identified; the arsonist gets a thrill witnessing the unfolding disaster). In the case of "medical terrorists"—those who would seek to kill patients in an organized fashion, often for political purposes—the option of being present or absent from the crime scene would remain open if poisons were given by way of the IV fluid bag.

COMMON, HARD-TO-DETECT MEDICINAL POISONS[1]

In Chapter one, a hypothetical scenario uses the common paralytic (muscle relaxant) agent called succinylcholine. Although certain tests in specialized labs can detect traces of this drug in the body (may take weeks to perform), this agent would never show up on routine toxicology testing because it is naturally broken down in the blood stream (and also, at places called neuronmuscular endplates) by a substance called pseudocholinesterase. Except in a very minute percentage of the population, which lacks this enzyme (so-called pseudocholinesterase-deficient patients), the drug is completely broken down to undetectable particles within about nine minutes. Unfortunately, if given rapidly enough—and in enough quantities—the drug will cause respiratory failure within thirty to ninety seconds; brain death is complete within six minutes. As we will examine in Chapter seven, there are deadly gases called "nerve agents," which have been used militarily in recent human history (for example, the two World Wars, and by Saddam Hussein against the Kurds as recently as the 1990s) to achieve the same results as succinylcholine. In quantities as little as five milliliters (one half of a standard ten cubic centimeter syringe), the colorless, odorless drug succinylcholine, given rapidly through an IV line (or injected intramuscularly), will more easily achieve the same deadly end as the nerve gases. Unless respiratory support is available immediately, patients will die from this medication. As mentioned, succinylcholine can also be administered by intramuscular (IM) injection, which would make it a particularly valuable drug for selective "assassination" in, say, a random—or planned—"injection stabbing". Succinylcholine will lose its potency if left unrefrigerated for anywhere from hours to days, depending upon the degree of warmth of its storage. Again, no secrets are being revealed in describing this common medicine, as we will later show that, unfortunately, now infamous health care workers have already used this drug to commit criminal acts.

Epinephrine (or adrenaline) is also a commonly occurring agent that exists in the body of every human being. Without it, we could not survive. This is the "fight or flight" endogenous (manufactured naturally in our bodies) drug that preserves heart rate and blood pressure, and opens our breathing passages. This is the wonder drug that is used in "epi-pens" (pocket-sized, self-administered, epinephrine dart) to treat severe allergic reactions (for example, a child with a bee sting allergy who has just been stung and is already swelling up and wheezing). Despite the common misinformation by dentists that their patients were "allergic to epinephrine" because their pulse raced after a routine dental injection containing local anesthesia plus epinephrine, there is no such thing as an epinephrine allergy. If an allergy to this compound were possible, those affected could never live within their own skin—this substance literally bathes every niche of our bodies at all times. The problem with epinephrine is that, if given in extremely high quantities to patients with unstable heart disease and/or pre-existing high blood pressure, it can cause a heart attack or stroke. Unfortunately, as we will see, real-life medical scenarios have already demonstrated how this drug has been used to kill in the health care setting.

Insulin is a drug used to treat diabetes. When used correctly, it keeps blood sugar levels from becoming too high, thus avoiding diabetic-induced, *hyper*glycemic comas. Although insulin rapidly loses its potency when warmed (must be stored in a refrigerator), it can be a profoundly deleterious agent if injected in high quantities either by IV line or by way of a shot into the skin or muscles. Longer onset and longer acting insulin medications can further separate the time interval between when the patient is "dosed" with the drug and when the drug actually takes effect. The reason why insulin can be so damaging is because high quantities can induce a dangerously low blood sugar level (*hypo*glycemia) that will result in total body shutdown, coma, and death. As a naturally occurring compound, insulin is also more difficult to detect with forensic toxicology.

This list of hard-to-detect medicines is incomplete, but it is not necessary to detail every type of potentially lethal drug on the doctor's shelf. The take-home point here is that all of these medicines are easily obtained/stolen/found in thousands of health care facilities across this country. As this book will later describe, these and other medicines are all too "available" and under predominantly lax supervision or storage security.

EASIER-TO-DETECT, EQUALLY ACCESSIBLE MEDICINAL POISONS

Local Anesthetics come in different types, and are readily accessible on most drug supply shelves. They are inexpensive and are used to numb tissues for surgery as well as to impart postoperative pain relief. Lidocaine is one variety of local anesthetic used to treat certain forms of cardiac arrhythmias (irregular heart beats). If administered in high enough dosage, however (even for legitimate, medicinal purposes, refer to Dorin's *Anesthesia in Cosmetic Surgery*, Chapter 8, Lidocaine Toxicity, editor Friedberg, Cambridge University Press, 2007), lidocaine can be deadly by causing heart block and heart failure. Bupivacaine is another, long-acting local anesthetic that can be lethal if misused. Bupivacaine binds to the proteins of the heart muscle itself, and can result in dangerously low blood pressure, irreversible heart failure, and death.

Other muscle relaxants that are longer acting than succinylcholine can create respiratory failure for an even more prolonged duration; in the absence of adequate artificial respiration, death will result. These can include the class of nondepolarizing neuromuscular blocking agents (for example, pancuronium, vecuronium, rocuronium, and atracurium). All of these muscle relaxants can be added to any conventional IV fluid bag without indication that the medicine is there. Virtually, every IV drug used for anesthesia, critical care, emergency care, or general medical purposes is without color, dissolves completely within any fluid medium (even if stored in a powder form), and is odorless. These medicines give no indication, whatsoever, that they have been administered until the therapeutic/physiologic effect takes hold.

Phenylephrine is a massively potent IV version of the over-the-counter drug neosynephrine. Phenylephrine, when used properly, can keep patients alive by supporting their blood pressure during surgery or during resuscitative efforts. The massive blood vessel constrictive effects of this medicine, however, can make it especially deadly if given in excessively high amounts to patients with pre-existing heart disease. It can also increase the risk of a cerebral vascular accident (stroke). Phenylephrine can cause cardiac failure in a weakened heart by creating such a massive constriction of blood vessels "downstream" from the heart that the pumping strength of this organ cannot overcome the resistance. The effect is as if the blood vessels are completely closed off and very little blood can reach the distal organs. By effectively shutting down the circulatory system, a massive dose of phenylephrine also starves the heart muscle itself.

All of the aforementioned drugs in this section are singled out because they are relatively inexpensive and abundant in clinical settings. Despite what medical administrators or government regulatory agencies would like you to believe, these medicines are not tracked closely and can be easily and deceptively "hidden" in conventional IV fluids to cause injury and death. The potential to cause great harm to multiple patients across multiple clinical settings exists. These examples (and that of the hypothetical scenario described in Chapter one) do not even presume tampering or conspiracy at the level of a manufacturer. All that is required is evil-minded or psychologically unstable individuals who are present in clinical facilities and who are willing to carry out such acts.

If we assume that there are other medical workers with the same sentiments as those foreign doctors who stood around the television set in my previous hospital operating room lounge (remember—those who cheered on 9-11-01 as they witnessed television footage of the carnage and murder), then the villains are already amongst us and we are already at a huge disadvantage. The individuals capable of carrying out the heinous act of poisoning medical supplies are likely already here, working in our American medical institutions.

Doctor Dorin's Remedy:

Two new medical innovations are required—both easily within our reach.

1. It would not take a great deal of imagination to devise and market IV fluid bags that are packaged and delivered in stronger outer plastic wrappings. The bags themselves should also be made with a cap on the injection port site. Additional replaceable caps should also be marketed to allow "resealing" of the bag's integrity after medicines are added to the bag.

2. A second innovation that absolutely must be recognized (and mandated) is the addition of a predetermined harmless dye (one of several distinct colors) to the vials of those medicines that could potentially cause serious injury or death in the doses packaged and used in the medical setting. For example, red could be assigned to the class of nondepolarizing muscle relaxants, and orange to succinylcholine; blue could be assigned to the class of potent drugs used to increase blood pressure, and so on. When these medicines are injected for normal medicinal purposes, the coloring would harmlessly dissolve in the blood stream. If these "color-marked" medicines, however, were injected into a bag of IV fluids (and there was no reliable indication—signature/note in the patient record—that the bag's purity had been purposefully violated by the practitioner), then the impurity would be grossly apparent and the bag could be immediately replaced.

Lastly, notice that the example of common medicines, which are capable of being turned into poisons (by injection into IV fluid bags or similar medical infusion containers), is only one simple example of how death can be delivered to innocent patients. Imagine, how the odds begin to stack against us—the "good guys"—when we also include other toxins that can be introduced to the medical arena. The topic of smallpox and anthrax infections or the use of conventional poisons (for example, cyanide) will be covered later in this book. Although these subjects are well covered in other texts, this book will briefly touch on bioterrorism and the vulnerabilities of health systems to agents of mass destruction.

The discussion of injuries caused by tainting normal supplies in the health care setting would not be complete without a brief mention of the scope of this problem. As subsequent chapters will detail, there are many more cases of health care crimes resulting in murder than we would like to accept. The newsreels of recent history abound in multiple examples, some of which we will mention. What is absolutely terrifying, however, is the notion that we are only seeing the tip of the iceberg. Specifically, I am referring to declarations by various health care gurus over the past ten years who have pushed for greater and more uniform standards pertaining to medical and nursing protocols. According to these analysts, the number of preventable deaths per year (in the

United States alone) in medical settings simply from iatrogenic origins (that is, errors) is greater than 100,000.[2] This author is postulating that a potentially large percentage of these preventable deaths is due to unknown (by accident or purposeful deed) drugs residing within seemingly "empty" IV fluid containers! In other words, if the two previous recommendations (contained within the Dorin's Remedy listed above) were fully implemented, we might very well see a decrease in the number of medical errors that result in serious patient injury. Furthermore, we would be taking a significant step forward in preventing medical murders and defending ourselves against organized attempts to inflict harm on a large scale.

COUNTERFEIT DRUGS

The World Health Organization estimates that counterfeit drug sales will reach seventy-five billion by the year 2010.[3] This is an area that has received significant attention from medical organizations the world over. In this country, such disparate agencies as the FBI, CIA, FDA, and ATF—along with various pharmaceutical companies—have come together to tackle this black-market industry. International illegal drug cartels have realized that they can turn greater profits (upwards of twenty to forty times greater), and be subject to lesser jail times if caught (usually six to twenty-four months) if they switch to "legal" medicinal compounds. In many cases, however, law-enforcement agencies have become aware that terrorist organizations are getting into the act to fund their other, more militant pursuits. This should be worrisome, because these organizations could easily—at any time—decide to unload purposefully tainted supplies.[4]

Counterfeit drugs could be "empty" packets of sugar; they could also be substandard productions of real medicines that lack the industry standards of efficacy testing, production safety protocols, and quality standards. These "fake" medicines are made to look like their brand and generic originals, but could also contain purposefully misleading labeling. The most frequently counterfeited medicines are those that are marketed to wealthy nations in the category of "lifestyle drugs" (for example, antihistamines, steroids, sexual enhancers). Other categories worldwide include AIDS, diabetes, cholesterol-lowering, and anticancer medicines. One can imagine that tampering with these medications cannot only induce injury by poison or deception, but also by the very act of omission. To a diabetic or AIDS victim, the absence of the proper drug to a treatment regimen can be lethal in short order. On the other extreme, it is reported that the FBI has picked up chatter between Al Qaeda cells describing a plan to double the dose of an ingredient in the common cholesterol-lowering medicine, Lipitor, in the hope of inducing liver failure in millions of American patients. Some estimates put the percentage of drugs sold over the Internet to American consumers, which are actually "fake" (even unwittingly from well-known manufacturers), at levels ranging from 30 to 85 percent.[5]

The topic of counterfeit drugs will be more fully described in a subsequent chapter, but the key point to make here is that medicines—whether real or counterfeit—are not properly tracked from legitimate factory source to the bedside. Clinicians rely on the label that is affixed to the drug they are administering. Doctors and nurses count on the packaging of IV fluids, and do not (and/or simply cannot) know if they are giving their patients a "pure" product (more on this point later).

PEERING INSIDE THE MEDICAL WORLD

To illustrate this point on a level more germane to my clinical profession, this would be an appropriate juncture to reveal a little-known fact about how anesthesiologists and nurse anesthetists practice in the operating room. This insight speaks well of the vigilance of these anesthesia providers, but is also telling in ways that are both ominous and chilling. Many anesthetic medications are produced in plastic or glass vials that contain a far greater volume of medicine than is actually needed for one patient. Due to cost-containment measures, many of these multidose vials contain preservatives, which allow them to be used for more than one patient. Although the practice of reusing multidose vials of medicines has, thankfully, fallen out of favor in recent years, it is still done. Since medicines should be drawn from their vials using aseptic technique, with clean needles and syringes, there is no reason why these medicines could not be used in more than one setting and for more than one patient. In fact, hospitals and surgery centers often have preprinted labels to affix to these medicine vials that show the date they were opened, the initials of the one who used them, and the last date the drug can be given safely for patient use.

The only problem is that most anesthesia providers will not use (or are uncomfortable using) a previously opened and labeled multidose vial of medicine. Some will explain their behavior and position by saying that they question the use of proper, "clean" technique by the previous user(s). At its face, this might sound like a very reasonable explanation—after all, the current clinician was not present when the vial was first opened and used. But those who practice anesthesia for a living have either experienced circumstances (or heard of the experiences of others) where things just didn't go right with a given patient. The typical story is one where a patient with no history of medical problems (who later undergoes lab tests that all come back "negative") has physiologic changes on the operating room table that are inconsistent with the surgical procedure or medicines given. Sometimes, the patient will remain paralyzed for many minutes or hours after all anesthetics are turned off; many times there is absolutely no explanation for the clinical picture that is observed. One can imagine that this sort of picture can make an anesthesiologist or nurse anesthetist look less professional or incompetent in the eyes of the surgeon and other operating room staff. It can also make for a bad doctor–patient relationship. The interesting point is that anesthesia professionals who experience these types of situations will often talk behind closed doors. It is not usual for someone to say something like "you know, I should not have used that opened vial . . . who knows what was in it."

Odd, isn't it that medical professionals will privately question the purity of medicines they use—and, indirectly, imply that the medicines they have given could have been tampered with?

Chance, Careless, or Criminal?

In the year 2000, studies indicated that between 44,000 and 98,000 Americans died each year from a cause other than the one they had checked into the hospital to fix; by the year 2007, some suggest this figure is likely to be well over 100,000 per year. Compare this number of deaths to the risk of dying from a commercial airplane flight (answer: you would have to fly nonstop for 438 years before crashing).[6]

3

EVIL PRECEDENTS—HEALTH CARE WORKERS GONE BAD

Knowledge speaks, but wisdom listens.

— Jimi Hendrix

...No one believes what she was saying. Someone was lying. The nurse had no explanation for why her patient went south, and yet she was the only person there. I was always suspicious of her. Maybe it was an innocent mistake and she didn't want to admit it. We'll probably never know. She's still working at the same place.

— Nurse practitioner

There are numerous examples of evil committed in modern times by health care workers against patients, spouses, and perceived enemies. These cases have been speaking to us from newspapers and television commentators for decades. Our challenge is to listen. A dangerous mistake would be to assume that the dark forces operating within men are limited to "one crazy person" or one isolated political cause. The capacity to do harm, to murder, lives within the unfathomable soul and knows no boundaries.

I once knew of a hospital administrator who was more concerned with covering up mistakes than confronting them. When he was approached with a disturbing pattern of patient injuries and death that were occurring in one department and under the care of one particular physician and nurse, he responded with a list of reasons why the hospital would not take action. First, he said, there was concern over a defensive lawsuit on part of the doctor because he was of a minority nationality. Second, it is said, he pointed out that firing the physician (who happened to have been "nonboarded" in his specialty) would set a "bad precedent" because "then we could lose the other nonboard-certified doctors from the medical staff." He went on to describe how a nurse had already been investigated for having affairs with several staff members and misappropriating hospital funds. But, he added, she could not be disciplined because he, as a hospital manager, had unknowingly "signed off" on her extracurricular activities and would ultimately be held accountable. As crazy as it might sound now, imagine how it felt to hear these words (as they were reported to me). All anyone in a position of authority in the health care field should do is to look for ways to improve the delivery of medical care and find innovative methods to minimize patient injury.

Subsequent meetings with this same hospital administrator brought to light the fact that the hospital had never created a system-wide "corporate compliance" manual to deal with such important issues as quality of care, employee discipline, billing/finance rules, and security regulations. In bold (I do not believe it was pure ignorance) defiance and violation of industry standards, as well as state and federal laws, this hospital had been literally flying by the seat of its pants—and unnecessarily placing its patients' lives at risk. It is profoundly frustrating to work with health care managers who put their own politics above the safety and security of patients and staff members. Health care is one area of our society where there is generally very little margin for error. Playing politics with health care carries with it so much more than one person's job or another person's ego; in the medical arena, poor judgment and an imprudent management style can result in a cascade of injury (and death) for literally thousands of people down the line.

We now live in an age where a stealth killer can (and very well may) stalk the corridors of our medical institutions—instilling fear and mayhem nationwide—much as the D.C. beltway snipers did back in 2002. Our world today is fraught with religious and ideological conflicts that frequently erupt into acts of terrorism against innocent nonparticipants. Recent history shows us that Islamic radicals have blown up civilians as they sat eating pizza in sidewalk cafes, as they shopped in commercial malls, and as they rode to work on subways; thousands have died because they showed up for work in high-rise buildings.

Various factions within Iraq have not honored the sanctity of the hospital in seeking revenge killings,[1] and U.S. intelligence reports have indicated that American hospitals are on the radar screen for attack by Al Qaeda cells.[2] Whether in the form of a dirty bomb or nuclear blast, or in the form of co-ordinated, individual attacks against American patients in health care settings, our nation is acutely vulnerable.

In June 2006, in the run-up to the comic/horror flick *Snakes on a Plane*, I was asked by an editor friend to fill in for her at an engagement that was to feature actor Samuel L. Jackson. I agreed, and was eager to meet this interesting movie star. A few days later, I was sitting next to him asking questions. I had already met the film's director, and the famed snake handler, Jules Sylvester. Now I was sitting face to face with the well-known celebrity of *Pulp Fiction* and *The Red Violin*, to name only a few of his films. Suddenly, I had the urge to ask a serious question—something that is often not well received by the rich and famous. Mr. Jackson was behaving amiably, so I thought I'd give it a try. My question was something like "how would you feel if the terrorist in your film gave an idea to the real bad guys—i.e., that of unleashing harmful animals,

toxins, or chemicals in an airplane flying at 30,000 feet?" I fully expected
an answer like "Hey, lighten up, it's only the movies"—or something like that.
Instead, Mr. Jackson said something else that gave me pause. As he leaned
over to pat my back, he said, "Adam, the lead bad guy is not a terrorist . . . he's
a gangster."[3]

The problem with today's modern society is that we are all so distracted
with the two extremes of life—the drudgery of work and negative headlines
on the one end, and the fantasy of high-tech entertainment on the other—that
none of us takes the time to survey the entire landscape to make sure we're
on sound footing, to insure that our basic safety and security needs are being
met. Such is the case with the institutions of modern medicine. Mr. Jackson
was entirely right; the movie's antagonist was not a terrorist at all but rather a
nasty gang leader who dealt in drugs and exotic, dangerous animals. But this
famous actor was also wrong, because a killer is a killer. The title describing
the bad guy did not matter. Both terrorists and gangsters use violence and fear
in unlawful ways to get what they want—and, oftentimes, innocents pay the
price for their actions. As a nation and a health care community, Americans
must look beyond superficial differences to glean insights into the minds of our
enemies. We cannot be distracted and look the other way, as did the previously
mentioned hospital administrator. We must heed the words of Jimi Hendrix
and listen to the wisdom that knowledge speaks. The following examples of
real-life health care workers "gone bad" set an evil, foreboding precedent.

THEY KILLED UNDER THE AWNING OF THE HIPPOCRATIC OATH

Since the mid-1970s alone, over three dozen American health care workers
(in and out of the hospital setting) have been implicated and/or convicted in
patient deaths.[4,5]

Robert Diaz was a nurse who worked at several health facilities in south-
inland county of Riverside, in California. Located east of the beaches of San
Diego and Orange counties, and covering the desert terrain leading to Palm
Springs, Riverside comprises mostly middle-class towns and farms that are far
more affordable than those in neighboring communities. It is not the type of
place where one would expect to see a string of medically related murders. Mr.
Diaz, a trusted member of the medical care team, killed twelve elderly patients
in 1981 by injecting them with large doses of lidocaine. He was convicted and
sentenced to death.

In 1984, the law caught up with Genene Jones, a pediatric intensive-care
unit nurse in Kerrville, Texas. She had been previously implicated in a number
of deaths on the pediatric hospital unit, and was finally convicted in the death
of a fifteen-month-old child. Her method of choice to dispose of her victims was
lethal injection of various powerful medicines; she was sentenced to ninety-
nine years in prison.

In 1987, a nurses' aide in Ohio and Kentucky was found guilty of killing
thirty-seven hospital patients. His name is Donald Harvey. He killed his victims

using suffocation, arsenic, and cyanide, and was sentenced to three concurrent life terms.

The year 1990 saw Richard Angelo, a nurse at Good Samaritan Hospital in West Islip, New York, convicted of three assaults and two murders. Mr. Angelo killed his patients by injecting them with intravenous (IV) paralytic drugs. He was sentenced to "fifty years to life" in prison.

Efren Saldivar killed his patients while presumably performing his duties as a trained respiratory therapist in California. He was born in Brownsville, Texas, and obtained his degree from the College of Medical and Dental Careers in North Hollywood. Beginning his job in 1988, working the night shift, Saldivar is thought to have killed more than forty patients (some believe it could have been as high as 120 patients) at the Glendale Adventist Medical Center. He was eventually caught and convicted of killing six patients in 1998. His drugs of choice were the IV muscle paralytics succinylcholine and pancuronium bromide (brand name Pavulon), and the opiate morphine. Six bodies that had not been cremated were exhumed; these demonstrated the muscle paralyzing compound pancuronium, which, unlike succinylcholine, remains intact in tissues for many months postmortem. Saldivar was sentenced to six consecutive life sentences without the possibility of parole.

In 1999, Orville Lynn Majors, a male nurse, was sentenced to three hundred years in prison for the deaths of six patients at the Vermillion County Hospital in Clinton, Indiana. Suspicion fell on the nurse when fellow colleagues and a supervisor noticed a higher death rate on his shift in the intensive care unit where he worked. An internal investigation revealed that, during the time of his employment, Majors was linked to one hundred thirty out of one hundred forty-seven deaths. The lethal potion of choice for nurse Majors was potassium chloride. If given in high enough concentration and rapidly enough, it will induce a deadly cessation of normal cardiac function. Potassium chloride is a naturally occurring substance in the human body. Occasionally, IV potassium must be administered to patients to bring blood levels into the normal range. This is done by giving low doses of the substance over an hour or more. There was time—not too long ago—when routine hospital drug carts contained potassium chloride for such a use. Unfortunately, there were serious errors nationwide due to the confusion caused by a dangerous similarity between the potassium chloride plastic vial and the vial used to contain clear, "normal saline" solution for IV patient use. The contents inside looked the same, and the packaging of the drugs was almost identical. Because of its ready availability at that time, potassium chloride would have been easily accessible to someone like Orville Lynn Majors. Presently, potassium is made less plentiful to bedside clinicians, being stored and prepared primarily in facility pharmacies, and then transported to the clinical floors in specially marked infusion bags.

Kristen Gilbert was a nurse, who in 2001 was convicted of killing four patients at the Veterans Affairs Medical Center in Northampton, Massachusetts. During her trial, it was shown that Gilbert enjoyed giving her lethal injections to patients because it resulted in a resuscitative "code" that allowed her to meet up with her boyfriend, a security guard. Gilbert received four consecutive life sentences for her murders. Her drug of choice was epinephrine (the naturally occurring compound, adrenaline).

Katherine Ramsland, Ph.D., who instructs in the area of forensic psychology at the University of Pennsylvania, has been quoted as saying health care serial killers are motivated by "human nature." She lists five types of "medical killers": mercy killers (kill out of compassion), those who kill for the erotic rush (physiologic "high"), those overburdened at work (motivated to decrease their patient load), those with a God-complex (a desire to dominate and control), and those who suffer from some other type of mental illness. Other workers in the area of forensic medicine have identified additional motivations for killing: contract killers (for money), those who kill under the influence of spiritual or charismatic leaders (cults, terrorists), power seekers (patients put at risk so the health care worker can "save the day" and be seen as heroic). Of course, the reality is that many killers will suffer from a host of ailments and delusions. One common characteristic of these types of murderers is that, to be successful, they must be well-educated, careful, and clever.

TELLTALE SIGNS OF A MEDICAL KILLER

Odd, isn't it, that medical schools spend more time teaching doctors how to spot the signs of drug addiction (so that colleagues can be referred to proper "rehab" programs and avoid losing their license) than they do teaching the telltale signs of a medical killer. I once knew a brilliant man who was the vice-chief of a major university residency-training program. On a personal level, he taught me some of the best clinical skills, which I use to this very day. This man, in fact, was so intelligent and accomplished that he was recognized the world over for his work. Unfortunately, he also suffered from a serious case of IV drug addiction. The doctor's habit was so strong that he would inject himself with the powerful opiate fentanyl (one hundred times more potent than morphine) while practicing in the operating room. All the signs of addiction were apparent and plain to see—the loss of weight, the frequent complaints of being cold, the wearing of long-sleeve shirts. One day, this doctor was found on the floor, in the corner of an operating room, unconscious and with a syringe stuck in his arm.

One would think that this would have been the end of this doctor's career. But nothing could have been further from the truth. He was sent to a state-sponsored, drug rehabilitation program, avoided the loss of his medical license, and was welcomed back to the "ivory tower" to work. Within a few years, he was granted the chairmanship of a department in another state.

I mention this example because it demonstrates the extraordinary lengths medical training programs will go to help their own—even when laws have been broken. Why, then, do physicians, nurses, hospital administrators, and health system attorneys look the other way when there are questionable signs (but, possibly, lack of absolute proof) of harm toward patients by health care providers?

The answer may surprise you. In fact, many of the signs (see below) of drug addiction are also seen in medical killers. The difference is that the medical profession sees a killer as a "defect" in the system, and system issues are notoriously difficult to treat. You can send a doctor or nurse off to a rehabilitation program, eliminating them from the clinical environment and hopefully fixing or mending the problem. If the system is wrong, people really have to scratch their heads to come up with explanations and solutions. Furthermore, when institutional "systems" are involved, multiple people may eventually be implicated—this is wholly unacceptable to the mentality of medical professionals. The last thing doctors, nurses, or hospital administrators want is to get embroiled in the legalities of accusing an employee of wrongdoing. And no one wants to see their dirty laundry displayed on the front page of a local newspaper. But there is really another, more disturbing reason why health care institutions prefer to look the other way when faced with unusual patient illnesses or deaths. It is because the system is so far "out of whack"—because so few safeguards are in place—that no one knows where to begin to solve the problem. Dealing with this issue must go far beyond the occasional editorial or article in a specialty trade journal; it must extend past the hospital boardroom. What is needed is a wholesale restructuring of the American medical system.

Some Warning Signs to Look for in the Workplace:

- Things tend to go wrong around the suspected individual.
- The suspect often works late shifts, when few colleagues are around.
- The suspect is known to "take" more medicine than is needed for the treatment of a given case.
- The suspect likes to work alone, has a history of abusive or failed relationships, and/or frequently makes unexpected, grandiose, or hostile statements about patients.
- The suspect is nonconfrontational and passive–aggressive.
- Accomplices to the suspect may be emotionally and/or sexually involved, and demonstrate an almost subservient deference to the suspect.
- Unexplained syringes or drug vials are noticed in the trash, hazardous waste bag, "sharp" container, or pockets of the suspect.
- Evidence of tampering or altering the patient chart is associated with the suspect.

In today's world of terrorism, we must also be willing to look at traditionally "personal" aspects of our coworkers' lives. Colleagues and health care managers must be willing to ask tough questions about a person's personal habits and life, if there is suspicion that a crime has happened or is about to be committed. In the struggle to prevent terrorist acts, there should be little patience for political correctness. It is possible to be kind, respectful, but blunt without encroaching on a fellow citizen's protected freedoms. If a person has nothing to hide, he or she should be willing to share their explanation of a particular act or event.

THE DARKEST SERIAL KILLER IN MEDICAL HISTORY

Sometimes, the most devious and deadly killers are the most difficult to detect. Harold Frederick Shipman (1946–2004) was a general practice doctor who lived and practiced in Great Britain. From the 1970s to 1998, it is thought that he killed approximately 250 patients. Most of his victims were elderly women who lived alone; many of them were previously in excellent health. Oddly, Dr. Shipman drew attention to himself when he attempted to pass a forged will in the name of one of his victims. He was convicted of fifteen counts of murder, but later committed suicide.

Shipman had been a respected member of the medical community. He worked as a general practitioner in Hyde, and founded his own medical clinic in 1993 on Market Street. In March 1998, Dr. Linda Reynolds of the Brooke Surgery facility in Hyde (just opposite of Shipman's clinic) went to the coroner for the South Manchester district with concerns about Dr. Shipman's practice. Something was wrong, she felt. After all, why were so many of his patients, otherwise seemingly healthy, dying? In particular, it was odd that Shipman had signed cremation forms for so many of these patients. Dr. Reynolds could not determine if Shipman's patients were victims of incompetence or malice.

The police began an investigation, during which time another three patients were found to have died. Initially, the police concluded that insufficient evidence existed to bring charges against Dr. Shipman or his clinic. The last victim of Shipman's practice had been the former Mayor of Hyde, Kathleen Grundy. She had been found dead at her home, and Shipman had been the last person to see her alive; he later put his signature to her certificate of death. A red flag was raised at the insistence of Grundy's daughter when a will was found that bequeathed 386,000 English pounds to Dr. Shipman without allotting even one penny to the daughter. Simple police work then "undid" the mastermind killer when Grundy's body was exhumed and found to contain levels of a high-grade, medical-type of heroin. A further investigation also detected that Shipman owned a typewriter with matching type to that used to create the forged will. A more complete investigation into the deaths of other patients also noted traces of morphine and medical records that had been altered or forged.

Some tried to psychoanalyze the motives of Dr. Shipman, who kept closelipped about his alleged criminal behavior. He vehemently defended the accusations against him, and sought to have the case of Kathleen Grundy (where money was seen as a motivator) separated from the other cases (where there was no perceived association with a motive, although stolen jewelry from other victims was later found in his garage). Many proffer that Dr. Shipman enjoyed the power he exercised over these women in controlling their life and death. Others have speculated that his actions could have stemmed from a deep-seated insecurity arising out of the death of his mother. The formal Shipman Inquiry even suggested that the doctor, himself, experimented with drugs.

Dr. Harold Shipman was found hanged in this prison cell the day before his fifty-eighth birthday, January 13, 2004.

MORE RECENT MEDICAL-RELATED MURDERS

In October 2006, Vickie Dawn Jackson, a forty-year old, former nurse, was sentenced to life in prison for killing ten hospital patients in Texas. Nurse Jackson decided to kill her patients—most of them hospitalized for minor, acute medical problems like diarrhea, foot sores, or dementia—because they were seen to be "too demanding." Jackson's lethal method of choice was to inject the respiratory paralyzing drug succinylcholine through her patient's IV lines.

On October 9, 2006, an emergency room doctor, Yazeed Essa of Cleveland, Ohio was arrested in Cyprus, Greece on charges of aggravated murder of his wife, Rosemarie Essa. Essa disappeared three weeks after the death of Rosemarie, having traveled abroad to places including Syria and possibly other Middle Eastern countries. Rosemarie called a friend on her cell phone gasping for air the day of her death, and said that her husband made her take calcium pills that were making her feel ill. It was discovered that Yazeed Essa was having an affair with a nurse. Essa's drug of choice for murder was cyanide that was laced in the contents of other calcium pills found in the same bottle used by Rosemarie.[6]

FROM TERRORIZED PATIENTS TO MEDICAL TERROR

It appears that federal and state agencies would like Americans to believe that medical-related murder is just that, an issue relegated to the files of law enforcement. Unfortunately, this attitude is wrong—and dangerous. It is likely that what is promulgated through the newswires, and offered as official advice, is also tainted by a desire to avoid public panic. To this end, terrorism against medical targets remains a "low threat"—low, that is, until the first large attack.

On June 10, 2005, the Department of Homeland Security issued a letter stating that hospitals are not specific targets of terrorist attack. The California Department of Health Services likewise faxed letters to 440 hospitals statewide confirming that "there is no information regarding any specific or defined" terrorist threat against state hospitals.

About that same time, however, FBI documents reveal that two men, Hamid Hayat and his father Umer Hayat, were arrested on charges of lying to FBI officials about their alleged involvement with a training camp run by Al Qaeda in Pakistan. In a seven-page affidavit, it is detailed that, after Hamid Hayat failed a lie detector test, he admitted to spending six months in an Al Qaeda camp where he was trained to "kill Americans . . . in the United States." The affidavit went on to state that "potential targets for attack would include hospitals and large food stores."

Days after the affidavit was released, the FBI retracted this last statement. They said that there had been a miscommunication, and that no threat against U.S. hospitals or food stores was present. When pressed by this inconsistency, *another* FBI agent was quoted as telling the *Los Angeles Times* that the risk of attacks against hospitals and grocery stores was deleted from the original affidavit because of concerns that the information might "panic the public."

The *Sacramento Bee* reported on June 10, 2005 that a homeland security bulletin was sent to California hospitals stating that "U.S. hospitals offer easy public access and would be recognized by terrorist planners as easy, accessible targets."[7]

See Appendix A for a thorough timeline of poisons, murders, and medical-related terrorism.

Chance, Careless, or Criminal?

Greater than 7,000 deaths per year in hospitals are estimated to be the result of "preventable" medication errors; this yearly number is likely to be more than double for the tens of thousands of additional nonhospital health care facilities. Half of the unexplained and adverse reactions to medicinal treatments are reported as medical errors.[8]

4

FAKING IT (COUNTERFEIT MEDICINES, CRIMINALS, AND TERRORISTS: THE HISTORY AND IMPLICATIONS OF COMPROMISED PHARMACEUTICAL SECURITY)

The safety and happiness of society are the objects at which all political institutions aim, and to which all such institutions must be...

—James Madison

...I know she was stealing drugs, and I proved it...Yeah, she got arrested, but I wish we knew what she was up to—I mean, where did the medicine go? Seriously, where did it go and who was affected?...and why?

—Pharmacist

THE SCOPE OF THE PROBLEM

The underground worlds of the illegal drug trade, counterfeit ("legitimate") medicines, terrorism, and international crime, all converge in a way that threatens the American consumer. Whether purchasing medicines over the Internet, buying drugs at the local pharmacy chain outlet, or being dispensed medication in a hospital, the risk of being poisoned or injured (from taking the wrong medication or an altered dose of the correct medication) is high.

To understand this vast, and often complex, area of pharmaceutical trade, we must first take a global perspective. The world of drug manufacturing and distribution is international; the immense scope of this commerce makes it especially susceptible to the entry of criminal elements. There is very little "testing" of medications by regulatory bodies, and hence the perpetrators give little attention to the accuracy and purity of their fake medications—choosing instead to focus on the appearance of pills, and packaging. On average, the cost to manufacture an illegal version of a legitimate drug may be less than one cent per pill in China or India, but this very same pill may sell for a quarter (or even as high as a dollar) in the United States. Even under the most attractive insurance "drug plan," twenty-five cents (or 2,500-percent profit) would likely still fall far below the cost of the real drug and be considered a bargain. In this way, "forged" drugs generate huge revenues for their criminal manufacturers. There is evidence to indicate that some involved in the illegal drug trade have switched their efforts to the area of counterfeit medications because of significantly lighter penalties in the event of capture and conviction.[1]

The U.S. Food and Drug Administration (FDA) and its counterpart in the United Kingdom, along with several other European nations, collectively agree with the following recent statement by the Royal Canadian Mounted Police: "Virtually all major organized crime groups are now involved in . . . counterfeiting pharmaceuticals."[2]

For decades, it was known that the Irish Republican Army used its illegal production of counterfeit veterinarian medicines to fund the purchase of weaponry. In November 2005, the U.S. House Subcommittee on Criminal Justice noted that "terrorists" were behind some of the anthrax scares that had been sweeping the country; in addition, the committee noted that intelligence sources were aware of terrorist funds coming from the Internet sale of fake drugs (e.g., ciprofloxacin to treat an anthrax exposure) as well as "chatter" indicating a desire to "spike" common drugs with deadly compounds. In March 2006, the U.S. Attorney Joint Terrorism Task Force unsealed an indictment charging nineteen people in an international terrorism crime ring that involved at least a half dozen countries. In a shocking revelation, it was disclosed that profits from the sale of counterfeit drugs were being wired to bank accounts used by Hezbollah.[3] In light of the Summer 2006 Lebanese War, and Hezbollah's open affiliation with the rogue regime in Iran, this information is all the more troubling.

The Internet has, unfortunately, become a haven for global profit centers in the areas of illegal online gambling, pornography, and pharmaceutical supplies. Almost everyone who has an e-mail account has received dozens—if not thousands—of spam messages selling sex and the "drug-du-jour" (the most common offenders are Viagra and the newer variations of the now-banned dieting supplement Ephedra). The Internet offers countless reasons to be attractive to criminals and terrorist organizations. One such example is that profits can be hidden via offshore tax havens and third world countries. Second, "mobile" and otherwise easily disguised operations can be hidden from law enforcement. Third, the components of a criminal network can be spread out so as to separate the big profiteers from the "street-level" of operations. For example, counterfeit copies of any given pill can be manufactured in China, but have a main Web address that is registered in the United States; having an American pharmaceutical title and corporate address (may only be a "dummy" post office box) gives a sense of false comfort to customers that they are purchasing a legitimate product. The scheme may utilize a European address for credit card payments, but process those payments in Indonesia. Usually, the data of other customers is used for the packaging return address. In this way, a confounding array of misinformation serves to distance the perpetrators from the day-to-day implementation of their crime.

The American public suffers from a relative lack of knowledge of the interplay between organized crime and terrorism. In fact, even the vast majority of practicing physicians are ignorant of the fact that as much as 85 percent of drugs purchased on the Internet, and even upwards of 30 percent of drugs bought in well-known pharmaceutical retail chains, may not contain the product they advertise.[4] There is a clear deficit of education regarding these issues amongst American health care providers. This author cowrote a short article (my wife, Shirin A. Dorin, D.D.S. contributed to the piece) entitled "Viagra and Terrorism," which was first rejected out of hand by several major medical journals for whom countless articles had been written over the past fifteen years. Their reason: "the information is not factual" . . . or, "if it's real, how come we don't know about this?" When I produced information from government sources, including the FBI, that supported the facts, there was an immediate change in the behavior of my editors. By then, however, my wife and I had already decided to place the article in our respective professional societies here in our hometown of San Diego. Both the San Diego County Medical Society and the San Diego County Dental Society were eager to share this information with their members in their monthly newsletters. The subject material was very well received.

The World Health Organization (WHO) Rapid Alert System, and the FDA Counterfeit Alert Network are two examples of provider notification systems that may help turn the tide in our fight to reign in counterfeit drugs. There is much work left to do, however, in making doctors, nurses, and patients aware of this problem. Part of the solution will be a sustained educational effort aimed at making people aware of the potential signs of fake drugs, and offering simple-to-use online forms for reporting suspected fraud.

A PNEUMONIC FOR SAFETY

One hero in the fight against counterfeit drugs is Dr. Bryan A. Liang, M.D., Ph.D., Juris Doctor of the Institute of Health Law Studies of the California Western School of Law and the San Diego Center for Patient Safety (University of California, San Diego School of Medicine). Dr. Liang originally developed the S.A.F.E.D.R.U.G. guide, which can be reviewed at the Web site http://www.safemedicines.org. An abbreviated version of this guide is as follows (the annotation here is provided by this author to better explain the acronym):

Sample: Obtain samples of the desired medicine from your physician; compare the taste, texture, appearance, etc. of the pill to that which may be later purchased from a land or Internet-based pharmaceutical company.

Appearance: Make a comparison between the drug and its packaging and a photograph of the legitimate drug in the Physicians Desk Reference (PDR). A copy of the current year's PDR can be referenced at most public libraries or online at http://www.PDR.net.

Feel: Be aware of the taste, sensation, and reaction you experience when taking the medication. Although legitimate generic versions of brand products may contain slightly different additives or preservatives, counterfeit drugs may have a completely foreign feel and taste from the original. Counterfeit drugs have been found with starch, saw dust, dry wall materials, and other seemingly unimaginable components.

Evaluate: Since counterfeit medications can contain no active ingredients, undesired or dangerous ingredients, or even too much medicine, it is important to carefully note what—if any—improvement is noticed with the use of the drug. *In the event of a serious side effect, notify your physician and pharmacist (and, if severe, go to the emergency room or call 911 immediately).*

Doctor: Make a point of following up with your physician, and take careful notes of your experience in the purchase, use, and reaction to the medication. Physicians and pharmacists are probably underused as partners in the fight against counterfeit drugs. These professionals have extensive connections with colleagues and their respective medical societies (both locally and on a national level). These contacts can help spread the word of problems rapidly so that others may potentially be spared the same experience.

Report: Your observations and experiences can be reported to the FDA at 1-800-FDA-1088, or on the Web at http://www.fda.gov/medwatch. Believe it or not, Federal officials really do "man" these Web sites and hotlines, and will take action to follow up on your concerns.

Unavailable: Remove the suspected medication from your personal medicine supply, and take it to your local law enforcement office.

Gather: Any additional information surrounding your use of this drug for further investigation; follow up with your physician to arrange to get the correct medicine as prescribed.

REAL-LIFE TRAGEDIES

In the early 1990s, several hundred children died of kidney failure in Nigeria, Haiti, India, and Bangladesh after a common syrup medication was laced with a toxic solvent.[5] Sadly, this event received little news attention in the developed world. Other examples, affecting predominantly impoverished areas of the globe, have been found in counterfeit versions of medicines used to treat typhoid, tuberculosis, and malaria. In an article of *The Lancet Infectious Diseases*, it was reported that nearly half of all medicines sold in Southeast Asia are believed to be fake. At the top of this list is a new antimalarial drug (artemisinin). In diseases such as malaria, where epidemic levels of suffering exist, there is little reason to think that expensive new agents will turn the tide of treatment successes with so much of the fake drugs flooding the market. November 2006 marked the new WHO initiative, International Medical Products Anti-Counterfeiting Taskforce (IMPACT), aimed at bringing together Interpol, customs officers, drug companies, and distributors to better tackle this problem.[6]

In the country of Niger, in 1995, over fifty thousand people were given a counterfeit vaccine for meningitis. The vaccines were supposed to have been from Pasteur Merieux and SmithKline Beecham. The fakes contained absolutely no medicinal ingredients that would function for their intended purpose.[7] Let us just pause and consider for a moment the consequences of giving a fake vaccine to tens of thousands of people. Not only were these vaccine recipients (or whomever footed the bill) duped into paying for something that could not possibly protect them, but they were put at risk from the vaccine injections of developing an adverse reaction to the ingredients; they, potentially, could have also acquired a viral or bacterial infection from dirty needles, inappropriate handling of the "vaccine," or tainted supplies. Finally, the recipients of the supposed vaccine were led to believe that they were protected from developing meningitis. Such a false belief could be incredibly risky to the extent that the "vaccinated" individual may feel more comfortable placing herself in harms way (e.g., working on a ward with known meningitis patients) or less inclined to seek treatment in the event the signs and symptoms of a meningitis-like illness were to appear.

Although the Chinese authorities were reluctant to release many details, it is known that 192,000 people died in 2001 after taking a "fake" drug.[8] The Chinese authorities, inclined to look the other way in cases of pirated or cloned electronic equipment, were forced to close thirteen hundred factories. In 2004, the Chinese discovered over twenty domestic manufacturers were putting counterfeit infant milk powder on the market. They closed the factories and arrested approximately two dozen people, but only after fifty infants had died.[9]

Some consider these and other tragedies difficult to combat in many non-Western countries, especially those in the third world. With limited resources, it would be unrealistic to expect these poorer countries to comply with strict regulations and testing. In America and other developed nations, however, it is unforgivable to consider *not* doing everything we can to prevent the loss of life associated with counterfeit drugs. To begin with, many have suggested strengthening the legal penalties for drug counterfeiting. This author suggests passing laws that allow sentences of greater duration (with no potential for parole; including the possibility of life imprisonment). Law enforcement officials should push for convictions and sentencing more consistent with those used for illegal drug traffickers. The tougher laws would increase prison time from the present guidelines of six months to two years (for counterfeiting) to twenty or more years (now, reserved only for narcotic trafficking); there should also be a mandatory forfeiture of assets and the assessment of treble damages to help offset the costs to society of pursuing and prosecuting these often complex legal cases.

Current technological advances such as Radio Frequency Identification (RFID) chips are only valuable as methods to track the packaging surrounding a given drug. One day, electronic sensors will be developed that can actually track individual glass vials of liquid medicine—and, possibly, the liquid, powder, or pills themselves. Technology has not yet advanced to this level, but more efforts must be applied to this area of research. Such measures would not only decrease preventable deaths, but would also decrease intrafacility theft and the diversion of sensitive medications within or between facilities.

A little known fact about medical personnel who work in multiple facilities in a given local region of the country is that medicines and medical supplies are often transferred between institutions. Sometimes, this is done inadvertently (e.g., in a bag or white jacket pocket), but also occurs out of convenience when a particular hard-to-obtain item is taken for later use. The problem with this behavior is that it can technically qualify as theft, and likely violates various accreditation, state and Federal rules about the handling of sensitive drugs and supplies. More importantly, however, is the fact that transferring medicines and supplies on ones person increases the possibility of loss, tampering, or damage (e.g., a vial of medicine left on a car seat, exposed to direct sunlight).

Sometimes, the counterfeited item is not a drug at all, but rather a medical supply or device. Such is the case with fake glucose test strips used by diabetics. On October 13, 2006, the FDA issued a warning to diabetic patients, alerting them to the detection of several phony blood glucose monitor test strips.[10] Multiple "lots" of fake strips were found to have been designed to mimic those manufactured by the Johnson & Johnson company. The phony supplies were for use with various models of LifeScan Inc.'s OneTouch brand of blood glucose detection machines. The LifeScan brand is owned by the Johnson & Johnson company.[11] The counterfeited strips could potentially yield falsely low readings, prompting diabetics to take too little insulin and other diabetes medicine (leading to *hyper*glycemia or high blood sugar; this can lead to organ damage, coma, and death). The illegal test strips could also lead patients to believe their blood sugar levels are higher than they really are, causing them to believe they need to take more medication. An inappropriately high dose of insulin, for example, can rapidly precipitate a dangerously low blood glucose level (or *hypo*glycemia). Severe hypoglycemia will present clinically as a profound lethargy, loss of consciousness, coma, and death. Although the FDA did not know how many lots of fake supplies were sold, they did issue data on the known counterfeited lot numbers. As a precaution, LifeScan voluntarily recalled other product line test strips based on preliminary sample testing that yielded inconsistent results. Since the manufacturer of the affected test strips distributed the items nationally via Medical Plastic Devices Inc. of Quebec, Canada and Champion Sales Inc. of Brooklyn, New York, the scope of serious complications from this breach of quality could have been extensive.

MORE REAL WORLD CASES

From the Archives of Homeland Security and the U.S. Customs Service.[12]

In 1986, David Jenkins (British silver medalist in the 400-meter relay at the 1971 Munich Olympic games), partnered with Juan Macklis of Tijuana to produce and smuggle steroids across the U.S. border.[13] In 1987, both Jenkins and Macklis, and over thirty others, were indicted in San Diego for this crime. Jenkins received a sentence of seven years in prison. Macklis remains a fugitive in Mexico, and is believed to be doing business under the banner of Victory Pharmaceuticals in Tijuana.

Javid Naghdi was extradited from the United Kingdom to the United States in 1989 for the crime of counterfeiting the popular antacid medication Tagamet. In 1990, Naghdi was convicted and sentenced to fourteen years in prison.[14]

In 1998, a couple was arrested at the Tijuana-San Diego border carrying bags of pills. An investigation revealed a trail that led back to eight Utah pharmacies. In 1999, three Utah pharmacists pled guilty for their role in buying substandard, counterfeited medications for pennies on the dollar from black-market sources. All three pharmacists went to jail and were forced to surrender their pharmaceutical licenses. The trail of fake drugs was believed to have traveled from India to Tijuana to Park City, Utah.[15]

In 1997, a patient died in Escondido, California from what was believed to have been substandard, counterfeited medication brought into the United States from Mexico. The offending physician, Dr. Castillo, was investigated by the FDA and the U.S. Customs Office; he pled guilty and sentenced to two years in prison, but escaped and fled to Mexico.[16]

In 1997, the FDA and U.S. Customs officials tracked down and seized twenty-eight million dollars in counterfeited medication produced in India. The medicine was stored in a San Diego warehouse, where it was discovered. One year later, pharmacists George Lopez and Christopher Kirkman were indicted; only Kirkman was prosecuted, and he received a sentence of only probation. The medication discovered at that warehouse was noted to be "filthy . . . and composed partly of dirt and sawdust."[17]

In 2004, the name of Juan Macklis (dba Victory Pharmaceuticals in Tijuana) resurfaced. It was discovered that approximately forty million dollars of fake Viagra tablets from India were being shipped to San Diego, destined for Tijuana pharmacies. The medicines would have eventually been resold to Mexican citizens and U.S. tourists. The drugs were confiscated at the border.[18]

WHAT PHARMACEUTICAL COMPANIES ARE DOING TO COMBAT COUNTERFEITING

It may be better to approach the subject of what pharmaceutical companies are doing to combat counterfeiting by addressing what they are *not* doing. In general, pharmaceutical companies appear to be doing very little to correct the roughly thirty-five billion dollars of fake drugs that reach consumers each year. Even though this figure represents a huge cost to American businesses, and eventually "hits" the consumer in the wallet, it is fair to say that cost alone is not nearly as important as the risk of disease or even death at the hands of impure or tainted medicines. The radio-frequency identification chips, as previously touched upon, cannot and will not be the only answer. This RFID chip concept may make better sense to those who have ever participated in an organized community race, such as a "10K" (ten kilometer), half-marathon, or marathon. Many of these running events use a similar electronic technology to track the athletes during every stage of the race. The computer chip allows for an accurate designation of where a runner is at any given moment, where he has been, and what route he has taken; the technology even knows if the runner has left the "grid" altogether.

Another way to track medications and supplies is to use the same bar-code/Wi-Fi electronic system commonly found in commercial mail carriers (e.g., UPS or Federal Express), or in big department stores and warehouses. Here, the bar code scanner takes inventory of the path a given product makes from one location to another; the Wi-Fi provides continuous, real-time data collection.

It is a simple, unfortunate fact that RFID chips are excellent at tracking cardboard—i.e., the "box" that carries the drug. And, RFID chips may be extremely valuable if used creatively in other areas of hospital security (see Chapters 5–7). The concept of electronically "tagging" and tracking medicine containers is a good first step, but unless we are able to literally follow the medicine itself, from factory floor to patient consumption, we are not making American consumers any safer!

To better understand this subject, we need to know what the U.S. FDA has done, and is doing, to protect the average consumer from counterfeit drug fraud. On a practical level, it is the pharmaceutical companies (who have hired their own investigators—many of whom will not disclose their identities and are former FBI agents), the U.S. intelligence community, and other national governments that are taking up this challenge. This problem, which is expected to reach seventy-five billion dollars in fraudulent business to worldwide consumers by the year 2010, is showing no signs of slowing down.

All the major U.S. drug companies have joined the act. The U.S. embassies in China, and other hotspots of drug counterfeiting such as India and Mexico, have patent specialists on hand to assist in trademark investigations. In 2005, the Chinese Vice Premier, Wu Yi, announced that China was cooperating with U.S. corporate offices to enforce international trade laws. In the late Summer of 2005, U.S. and Chinese authorities launched *Operation Cross Ocean* on tips from Pfizer and Eli Lilly & Co. The intention was to thwart the illegal production of Viagra's active ingredient in Central China (packaged in the Chinese port city of Tianjin and then shipped to the state of Washington). The pills were shown to contain poor quality control and consistency, and have upwards of 132 percent of Viagra's active ingredient, sildenafil citrate. This international law enforcement effort netted 4.3 million dollars in counterfeit Viagra. Fake Cialis (similar male sexual enhancer) and Lipitor (used to lower high cholesterol) pills were also seized. Twelve individuals were arrested.[19, 20]

At the time of the cooperative Chinese-American effort, John Theriault worked as the vice president of global security for Pfizer. Theriault's resume was replete with experience as a veteran FBI agent. He and others from various nations have joined big business in fighting the scourge of fake drug manufacturing and trafficking. With the growth of globalization, the ease of Internet communication, and the ability to evade authorities by hiding operations in remote locations across the Earth, it is a positive sign indeed that so many nations and companies have begun to work together to fight this problem.

One of the motives for these joint efforts, of course, is the simple economic challenge to legitimate companies. Another motive invokes the moral imperative to protect the well-being of innocent consumers. Using only the simple example of Viagra, it is well known that high levels of sildenafil citrate can cause serious cardiac complications and even death.

The major drug companies in the United States, such as Abbott, Merck, Pfizer, and Eli Lilly & Co., have also hired local personnel to infiltrate the networks of foreign counterfeiters. Utilizing people who speak the native language has facilitated undercover sting operations. Nevertheless, the criminals have become increasingly sophisticated and penetrating their organizations has met with only mixed success.

In February 2004, the FDA issued the report *Combating Counterfeit Drugs: A Report of the Food and Drug Administration.* The report highlighted the following areas for improvement: increasing international law enforcement cooperation and penalties for counterfeit perpetrators, heightened government vigilance and enhanced regulatory oversight, and better measures of drug packaging and tracking as medicines move through the U.S. commercial distribution chain. In 2004 alone, the FDA's Office of Criminal Investigations initiated fifty-eight separate surveillance and law enforcement cases—up from just thirty cases the year before. Reportedly, the number of such cases has increased each subsequent year—something that speaks well of the FDA's commitment to fighting drug counterfeiting, but also begs the question of how deep this criminal "iceberg" extends below the surface.[21]

Legitimate Generic Drugs Are O.K.

It is important for the consumer to understand the difference between potentially compromised drugs (e.g., tainted, counterfeit) and legitimate generic drugs which are manufactured by trusted pharmaceutical houses here in America and abroad. Once a brand drug goes "off patent," other companies can apply to the U.S. FDA for permission to manufacture that same medication and market it to the public. Generic medicines (both prescription and over-the-counter) usually hit the drug store shelves at a wholesale cost of anywhere from 30 to 70 percent off the brand name product. If the original pharmaceutical company is still producing the original drug, they will often make a huge marketing investment trying to convince the consumer that their brand is superior to the generic "knock-off". There is no across-the-board evidence to support that these claims of superiority are valid.

Generic medicines are cheaper because the laboratory making them does not need to recoup huge research and development costs; furthermore, these generic manufacturers do not spend nearly as much money advertising their products (if the drug itself is already popular, shoppers will be on the lookout for the less expensive version of the drug).

It is important to know that every generic medication must be individually approved by the FDA. Generic drugs are required to contain exact quantities of the same *active ingredients* (in the same dosage form) as the original product. The Drug Price Competition and Patent Term Restoration Act (September 1984) is responsible for the current availability of most generic medicines. This Act streamlined the generic approval process by decreasing paperwork and applying better-defined standards for equivalency between the new and the original drug. Some of the requirements for generic drugs include the following: The drug must have the same chemical formulation; the drug must have the same therapeutic effect; the drug must be bioequivalent (i.e., have the same qualities/effects in the body); the drug must meet FDA standards for purity, quality, stability, and strength; the drug must have the same labeling as the original brand medicine.

Hospitals and other health care institutions today are looking for better ways to keep tabs on their valuable products. One such solution is the automatic supply and patient tracking software of Patient Care Technology Systems (a subsidiary of Consulier Engineering, Inc.).[22] This product touts the ability to track equipment and patients for up to a thirty-five operating suite department. The company's business has been growing because of the increasing desire by facilities to "locate, track and orchestrate the flow of patients, staff and mobile medical equipment in order to streamline care, improve patient safety and optimize department management."[23] The company claims that its product works with all "locating" technologies, to include Wi-Fi, RFID, and infrared systems.

Ultimately, technology will make a difference in not only thwarting terrorism and criminal acts in general, but also in improving the quality of the medicine we deliver. Technology can indeed save lives in more ways than one. Nowhere is this better demonstrated than in the neonatologist, Dr. Chris Lehmann of Johns Hopkins University Hospital.[24] He has devised integrated computer technology systems that allow medical care to be delivered safer and more efficiently. Lehmann helped write a software program that quickly compiled and organized essential patient data to facilitate the daily progress notes physicians had to write on their patients. He also put together a guide to emergency resuscitation for babies that automatically calculates doses based on weight and other known physiologic parameters. His team's efforts have reduced errors over 90 percent by electronically calculating intravenous line "drip" rates; the Hopkins group also found an effective method to reduce errors in medication ordering through computer technology.[25]

It is clearly a sign that times are changing when the *New York Times* gets into the act. In February 2007, it ran a piece describing the horrible consequences of fake antimalarial drugs flooding into poor, third world countries.[26]

These counterfeit medicines (some composed entirely of fillers; others with only acetaminophen to reduce fevers or possibly a reduced dose of the stated drug) have been associated with upwards of hundreds of thousands of deaths per year. According to WHO statistics, 200,000 of the roughly one million malarial-related deaths per year could be prevented if patients were receiving the real medication. The *New York Times* identifies China as the largest source of counterfeit drugs worldwide.[27] If you walk into a pharmacy to buy an antimalarial drug in Southeast Asia today, you have a 53 percent chance of getting a fake instead.[28]

The FDA report sets a target year of 2007 for the realistic implementation of creating electronic "pedigrees" for drug production and shipping via RFID technology. In the year of this book's publication, however, there is little use of this technology nationwide. Despite the FDA's good intentions to foster the use of electronic product codes (EPCs) and other forms of electronic serial numbers, the technology still faces major financial and practical hurdles. As stated, the radio frequency chips are only capable of being tracked at a distance of a few meters; furthermore, they only track the drug packaging itself—something that can be easily circumvented by clever counterfeiters. Real, long-term benefits in this area will rely on ongoing efforts to develop drug dyes and chemical markers that actually exist within the medicine itself. This technology will require a system of planned and random testing sites along the path from factory to bedside. Not mentioned in the FDA report, or subsequent governmental reports for that matter, is any evidence that regulators are pushing for more precise drug tracking mechanisms. In this author's view, there must be a major, federally supported research and development push to utilize nanotechnology as a means of tracking the integrity and purity of actual drug components. Until this occurs, all drugs will remain vulnerable to large-scale counterfeiting and manipulation by terrorists and other criminal groups.

Chance, Careless, or Criminal?

The Institute of Medicine has estimated that preventable medical errors cost the American economy seventeen billion dollars per year. In a survey by the American Society of Health-System Pharmacists, 61 percent of Americans responded that they were "very concerned" about being given the wrong medication.[29]

5

HOSPITAL AND SURGERY CENTER "SECURITY" . . . OR LACK THEREOF, PART I: OVERVIEW

> The superior man, when resting in safety, does not forget that danger may come. When in a state of security he does not forget the possibility of ruin. When all is orderly, he does not forget that disorder may come. Thus his person is not endangered, and his States and all their clans are preserved.
>
> —Confucius

> . . . When I came back after lunch, I noticed that my narcotics were missing. I locked my cart—or at least I thought that I did. I think it was the surgical technician who stole them, but I can't be sure. Frankly, it's my fault. I know we're not supposed to carry the drugs around, but I should have kept them in my pocket."
>
> —Anesthesiologist

Physicians, nurses, and other health care workers are, at their core, scientists. Regardless of their background or religious tendencies, they are people who share a common personality trait—i.e., they strive to arrive at the truth, the origin, or cause of a particular phenomenon or disease. This is an admirable and necessary trait for those whose daily work involves decisions and actions that turn, fundamentally, around the hope for healing and the ever-present potential for injury. It is the health care provider, alongside the myriad of other technical specialists in today's modern society, who navigate life through the application of the "scientific method." The scientific method is based on observation, testing, experimental "treatments," and the notation of changes in our observations as a result of our new interventions. Whether we are aware of it or not, most Americans live their lives in a constant theater of data, numbers, and statistics. We are so inundated by this scientific underpinning to the decisions we make (e.g., buying a car, choosing a snack food, deciding which medication to take to lower our blood cholesterol, etc.), that we have become psychologically dependent on the need for information (data) to support almost all of our decisions.

The rigorous thinking and analysis that qualifies and quantifies our twenty-first century thinking is also the very thing that holds us back—that prevents us from seeing the broader, more abstract picture. Einstein was a genius and a definitive man of science, but when he took the exponential leap to envision a new view of the Universe (as just one example, seeing gravity as a distortion of the space–time continuum, not merely as a measurable, Newtonian force), he was exercising intuition, creativity, and imagination—not the rules of science. In fact, it was after much scorn and public repudiation, and many years later that Albert Einstein received the scientific confirmation (and world recognition) that his theories of special and general relativity were, indeed, correct. Such is the challenge of our generation to rise above politics to see the very real threat of terrorism to the American infrastructure, and to formulate methods to better secure our people. There is very little known in the public consciousness about the vulnerabilities of our health care institutions to terrorism. As in the days before 9/11, when there was no community awareness or large-scale questioning of airline security protocols, we are in waiting of a storm that will inevitably hit the shores of our medical system. The signs and history of "attacks" against health care targets are all there for us to see, if we choose to do so; we *must* choose to do so! Other than the facts presented thus far in this book, we will need to rely on our observational skills—and intuitively extrapolate these observations—to arrive at meaningful conclusions about the weaknesses of our health care facilities. First we must survey the larger canvas that is the modern, civilian American hospital or surgery center; then, we must begin to think like a terrorist so that we may know our enemy.

Today's hospitals and surgery centers are designed to allow a comfortable flow of people (providers and patients) in and out of places where medical care is delivered. From the architectural blueprints, to the various technological necessities, our medical institutions are made to facilitate the ingress and egress of visitors, family members, patients, and health care workers in as smooth a fashion as is reasonably possible. Sometimes, there are barriers to the free movement of individuals or supplies (e.g., receptionists, electronic cards that open doors, locks on cabinets), and sometimes employees will themselves notice unusual activities or unfamiliar faces, but the state of medical security in the United States is pathetically lax. In most hospitals and surgical centers, it is easier to enter restricted areas, steal, plant, and/or tamper with supplies than it would be to shoplift in the neighborhood department store.

THE HISTORY IS THERE IF WE CHOOSE TO STUDY IT

Isn't it odd that in our post-9/11 world we should choose to ignore facts that implicate the extremely lax degree of security in American medical institutions? Are we suffering from a case of "Iraq War" overload, where the only acceptable treatment is a self-administered dose of denial? Do we really believe that our suppression of reality—and our state of indifference—will protect us from attack against relatively helpless victims in hospitals, surgery centers, and other health care facilities? Maybe, we've just had enough and don't have the energy or resources to muster an adequate defense. But why, then, is it obvious that our own government is acutely aware of each and every risk outlined in this book and simply chooses to withhold this information from the public—is it simply out of fear that a panic will develop? Possibly, our elected officials and other civil servants are acting out of a noble attempt to balance community safety against the stability of our commercial markets. If true, it would be sad that our own representatives do not trust those who have put them in office with the very information that is necessary to protect all of us.

In late April 2005, the FBI and local law enforcement officials were called to look into suspicious incidents in Los Angeles, Boston, Detroit, and Sussex County, New Jersey, in which unknown individuals were found in protected and restricted areas of three hospitals. Evidently, the suspects were caught posing as inspectors for the hospital accrediting body, the Joint Commission on Accreditation of Healthcare Organizations (JCAHO). In all of the incidents, the "imposters" were actually stopped by security guards and staff members, but only after they had been on the grounds for an indeterminate period of time. There is no evidence that any of them were detected by conventional video-monitoring technology that is widely available and routinely used to pick out shoplifters in most large retail stores. There is no way of knowing how long these individuals were on the premises, or what information they took away with them. Very little is known about these intruders because none of them were arrested or questioned; their identity was never ascertained as they were simply asked to leave.[1]

Shortly after these fake hospital accreditation surveyors were detected, Brain Roehrkasse, a Department of Homeland Security spokesman gave a statement that flatly denied any intelligence information indicating that Al Qaeda—or any other known terrorist group—was planning an attack against American medical targets.[2]

The JCAHO is a respected—if not occasionally embattled—organization charged with the task of surveying and accrediting all U.S. hospitals. As will be addressed in Chapter 8, this organization and other accrediting bodies also survey private medical facilities and surgery centers. Most state governments as well as the new Federal medicare establishment, the Center for Medicare and Medicaid Services (CMS), also have bureaucracies that conduct surveys of medical establishments, clinical laboratories, and other treatment facilities to insure a basic minimum level of clinical care and compliance with regulatory statutes. As it turns out, and for good reason, some of these surveyors are expected to arrive "unannounced" to avoid the tendency for facilities to artificially "ramp up" their performance and disguise their true activities prior to a known accreditation survey. Once present on a medical campus and upon disclosure of credentials, individual surveyors can ask to see confidential patient records, observe work habits, gain access to restricted patient care areas, ask for keys to unlock drug repositories, and see detailed blueprints and schematics of facility layouts. Presumptively, the architectural blueprints are used to assess compliance with fire code requirements, make sure certain "medical building" standards are met, and ascertain that patient care is provided in a safe and reasonable fashion. These surveyor organizations can also interview employees and gain intimate details of an institution's inner mechanisms and security protocols.[3]

In the first hospital-imposter case, a man and woman (evidently very well dressed), were stopped in a Los Angeles hospital at about 2 a.m. They flashed badges similar to those used by JCAHO employees, but the timing of their arrival sparked suspicion and they were denied entry to the hospital by the security guard.[4] Keep in mind that, had they simply chosen to enter the hospital lobby during normal daytime hours, they would have met with no resistance or suspicion. This fact is abjectly obvious to anyone who has ever entered a community (nonmilitary) hospital to visit a patient.

Three days later, a second incident occurred at a hospital in Boston, where another well-dressed gentleman was seen trying to gain access to a hospital. This individual was middle-aged, and thought to be of Middle Eastern or possibly South Asian descent. He was also noticed in the early morning hours, at about 3 a.m. The man came across with some degree of authority. When asked for proper identification, however, he fled the facility.[5] The third episode occurred on the maternity ward of a Detroit hospital, where a woman identified herself as a JCAHO surveyor, but later fled when her behavior became suspicious to staff members. Again, it is not known how much information the individual gained prior to the heightened scrutiny of her presence on the locked ward.[6]

In late March 2005, in an incident quite different from the others, three men approached a security officer in a Sussex County, New Jersey hospital and identified themselves as doctors. They then asked for a hospital directory and detailed information about the institution's medical services and bed capacity. In response to this cluster of four suspicious cases, the JCAHO sent out two alerts to its roughly five thousand member institutions apprising them of the incidents and asking them to be more vigilant to potential intruders. Unfortunately, Federal officials chose to offer no further insights into these events. The Joint Commission simply updated its security procedures, indicating that surveyors will now carry a signed letter by the JCAHO executive vice president.[7]

In the Fall of 2005, Senators Barbara A. Mikulski and Paul S. Sarbanes (both D-Maryland) announced that both bodies of Congress had given final approval to the 2006 Department of Homeland Security Appropriations bill. This was an important first step for hospitals and other high-risk nonprofit institutions, giving twenty-five-million dollars in "seed" money toward better protection against terrorist attacks aimed at these most vulnerable of social institutions. More importantly, it was an acknowledgment at this highest level of government that American health care was acutely vulnerable to terrorism. In the aftermath of the September 11, 2001 attacks in New York and Washington, D.C., there has been significant activity on the part of medical personnel in organizing teams to combat chemical and biological terrorist attacks. Sadly, there has been little, if any, work done to shore up weak systems in place to prevent these and other attacks in the first place. One early exception has been the University of Kentucky Chandler Medical Center, which, in the Spring of 2004, announced its plans to implement a perimeter security system around the medical campus. This new system of protection would better protect students, staff, faculty, patients, and visitors by implementing a layered approach to security protocols and limiting access to public entrances.[8, 9]

A Brief History of "Bioterror"

It is evident that direct and "real" threats against American medical targets that exist from radical, political groups (e.g., Islamic fundamentalists) remain predominantly a mystery to the lay public. Understandably so, this type of information should remain within the confines of our intelligence community; its release could jeopardize ongoing investigations. Nevertheless, we have already shown some of the vulnerabilities, which exist to patients at the hands of "crazy" health care workers and others, and it would behoove us to take a look at those weaknesses which have existed (and do exist) within the realm of American health care from all potential sources. A component of this evaluation will require us to examine bioterrorism and what is being done to better prepare (and support) our nation in the struggle against potential, future attacks. Although this text is not specifically concerned with the methods of identifying and treating chemical, biological, or nuclear attacks against civilian populations, we should be concerned with all of them.

Government contacts who request to remain anonymous have confided to this author that more is being done to protect our citizens in the area of health system security than may readily meet the eye. For example, the government (as coordinated via the Department of Homeland Security) has set up several "test sites" to analyze real-time data from retail pharmacies and emergency rooms in an attempt to detect "spikes" in unusual behavior, injuries, infections, and drug use. Two of the test sites were revealed to be in the Washington, D.C./Northern Virginia/Suburban Maryland metropolitan area and the San Diego area. The goal is to see if computers and human analysts can decipher reams of "live" data to pick up evidence of criminal and terrorist activity, or early tips that a biological weapon may have already been released into the general population.

The Institute of Medicine of the National Academies, in its June 2006 report brief, described what it deemed significant as deficiencies in this country's ability to respond to a natural disaster, pandemic, or terrorist attack.[10] The report goes on to describe how the nation's inadequate hospital emergency response preparation, capacity, and training will render communities woefully "at risk" should a major disaster occur. As explained in the report, much of the problem could be properly addressed with increased funding. In 2002, the government Bioterrorism Hospital Preparedness Program doled out only five to ten thousand dollars per selected emergency services department. In 2002 and 2003, emergency departments and providers received only 5 percent of the Bioterrorism Hospital Preparedness Program's funds, and only 4 percent of the nearly 3.5 billion dollars distributed by the Department of Homeland Security.[11] The report continues to explain that most hospitals lack the proper tools necessary for even a basic response to a disaster. As a further example, most medical institutions do not have the specialized isolation units required to contain, treat, and prevent the spread of deadly airborne virulents.[12]

BRIEF BIOTERROR HISTORY[13, 14]

Let's briefly examine bioterrorism in an attempt to better understand the "soft spots" inherent to our free and open health care system. Bioterrorism is the use of viruses, bacteria, fungi, and organic (or organically produced) compounds to poison other living creatures (i.e., humans, other animals, and plants). Bioterrorists can be homegrown or foreign; they can represent local interests (e.g., reactionary, bigoted militia groups) or international hate movements (e.g., Islamo-fascists bent on killing Christians, Jews, and other representatives of western society). In all cases, the use of terror is a potent tool to instill fear and send a message that our way of life is vulnerable to disruption and destruction.

Although one could argue that terrorism is merely another variant of war, and that mankind has been at war since our earliest days on this planet, there are historical milestones that can be traced in the recorded tales of man's attempt to kill his brother. Starting with Cain and Abel, murder has been a regular staple of human endeavor. But biological warfare or terrorism may be dated to the fourteenth century, when the city of Kaffa (located on the Crimean Peninsula) is thought to have been deliberately targeted with plague. It is thought that competing merchant "gangs" on the ancient silk route between Europe and China made war against the Tartar tribesmen. It was believed that the tribesmen carried the plague from eastern provinces. Both sides were known to have used (e.g., catapulted over walls and fortresses) infected corpses as weapons.

Historians have noted that the British took scabs from suspected smallpox lesions of sick patients and littered them in blankets, clothing, and other items in an attempt to infect enemy Indians during the eighteenth century. World War I saw the use of mustard gas as a weapon. During World War II, in 1943, the United States learned that Japan had developed biological weapons; that same year America itself began a formal biological weapons program. By 1953, the U.S. Department of Defense had begun a sophisticated biological warfare program at Fort Detrick, Maryland. Despite President Nixon's signature to a treaty banning biological weapons in 1969, it is known that deadly biological agents (and samples of chemical toxins) are kept preserved in multiple laboratories and other government facilities throughout the United States.

Biological "agents" used to kill offer many advantages over other methods of mass murder. In many cases, rogue laboratories can produce the agents with a fair degree of safety and at a low cost. Infection can be delivered through indirect methods to introduce the agents to the skin, mucous membranes, and lungs (e.g., via aerosol spray, ventilation systems, etc.), and hence distance the perpetrator from the crime by space and time. In the case of true infections—as opposed to biological toxins—the population at large then acts as a perpetuating source of new infections, illness, and death. Once a large epidemiological diagnosis is made as to the nature of the offending agent (and as to the suspicion of terrorism), treatment is complicated and often faces difficult, logistical hurdles. Public panic is often a desired outcome of the terrorists in such scenarios. Treatment can also be expensive, and the morbidity and mortality rates of biological terrorism are likely to be high. Even when biological terrorist threats are determined to be fake (i.e., a hoax), an element of fear, disruption, and social unrest nevertheless scores a victory for the bad guys (e.g., 1999 alone saw almost eight hundred separate cases of "anthrax scares" in America).

The U.S. Federal government lists the following as potential agents of biological terrorism:

- Variola major (smallpox)
- Eastern equine Encephalitis
- Botulinum toxin
- Ricin
- T-2 Mycotoxins
- Bacillus anthracis (anthrax)
- Yersinia pestis
- Brucella spp
- Francisella tularensis
- Vibrio cholerae
- Coxiella burnetii (Q-fever)
- Viral hemorrhagic fever
- Staphylococcus Enterotoxin-B

In the past three decades, we can look to eight significant worldwide "bioterrorist" events to better appreciate what evil minds have done (and can do) to disrupt the lives of innocent people. In 1979, in Sverdlovsk, Russia, a government military facility specializing in biological warfare fell victim to what U.S. intelligence sources described as a lapse in security and poor handling techniques. It is reported that both civilian and military fatalities occurred to the toll of hundreds of victims. The lethal agent was anthrax—spread through the air, with the initial symptoms being that of pulmonary infection.

In 1984, in Oregon state, a cult of Rajneesh followers contaminated local salad bars in the city of Dalles. Their agent of choice was Salmonella; their hope was to influence a local election by creating a large body of citizens who were too sick to make it to the voting polls. In all, 751 cases of Salmonella poisoning occurred. To confirm their case, the Oregon police and department of health presented evidence that the Rajneesh had grown genetically identical cultures of the infecting organism in a secret laboratory.

The year 1994 in Tokyo, Japan, saw the now infamous subway attack of innocent civilians by the Aum Shinrikyo cult group. The Aum Shinrikyo used sarin gas as their agent of death; their attacks resulted in eight deaths, with another roughly one thousand victims falling ill (about fifty of them seriously ill). An additional four thousand subway travelers were evaluated for potential signs of illness in local hospitals. In all, a great commotion and state of unease was created by the terrorist actions of this deadly Japanese group.

In the mid-1990s, the FBI investigated several anthrax threats that occurred throughout America. In 1995, in Arkansas, a threat of Ricin toxin was revealed to be a hoax. In 1996, in Dallas, Texas, an employee of a large medical laboratory laced pastries in the employee lounge with cultures of Shigella. The contaminated food resulted in twelve severe cases of dysentery requiring hospital care. The late 1990s saw the anthrax hoax against a Washington, D.C. B'nai Brith headquarters (1997). Subsequent anthrax attacks in the United States resulted in injury and death. The late 1990s and early part of the twenty-first century also saw a slew of anthrax (or fake, white powdery substances) sent via the U.S. postal service to various public figures and members of the U.S. Congress.

If we amended the previous list of biological terrorism agents to include toxins, we would have to include the following entities: Abrin toxin, Aflax-toxins, Botulinum toxin, Shiga toxin, Saxitoxin, Ricin, Diacetoxyscirpenol, C. perfringens (Epsilon toxin), and Conotoxins.

The following two chapters will examine "inside" information on the vulnerabilities to attacks against U.S. hospital/medical facilities that exist from those wishing to do us harm from external as well as internal, vantage points. First, however, we should further explore the general condition and history of our national hospital system's state of readiness to dealing with terrorist threats.

It is human nature to try to deal with threats to our very lives by "reacting"— i.e., by finding ways to both avoid risks and deal with the consequences of disasters once they have struck. It is also human nature to weigh the costs (time, expense, and personnel) as well as the benefits, and come down somewhere in a middle ground where we have at least satisfied our need to "do something." Unfortunately, in the case of terrorism, simply "doing something" is not enough. The various community projects to amass medical personnel, police and firefighting professionals, and medical experts are necessary measures in preparing to treat chemical, biological, or other deadly attacks against civilians. These steps will require supplies to treat various injuries, neutralize toxins and caustic agents, and protocols for the quick establishment of mobile triage and treatment units. Alas, none of these measures will be adequate in containing and effectively treating attacks if they occur within the boundaries of medical facilities themselves. This will be especially true if the attacks are well coordinated and involve several hospitals or similar facilities in a given geographic location.

BACK TO THE MODERN RECORD OF HOSPITAL IN-SECURITY

On March 19, 2003, three men arrived at the emergency room of Southwest Regional Medical Center in Little Rock, Arkansas. The individuals were dressed in military uniforms and generated some degree of suspicion, most particularly when they announced that they had been assigned to that location to protect the hospital against some unspecified attack. The individuals disappeared as quickly as they had appeared; later it was discovered that no military unit had been assigned the duty of protecting Southwest Regional's emergency room. The FBI was reported to have investigated the incident, but no specific follow-up or findings were ever announced. In two other cases involving Midwestern hospitals, some people had arrived offering to specifically and exclusively volunteer to work in the boiler room area. The two hospitals turned the individuals away because they did not need volunteers for that location of their physical plant. Unfortunately, it was much later that hospital administrators realized their mistake in not reporting such strange volunteer requests to authorities immediately. No successful follow-up was ever made to determine who the inquiring individuals were, or if they were acting nefariously in concert with others.[15]

Hospitals "operate" by being relatively fluid and easily accessible to staff, patients, and visitors during most hours of the day. Usually, various personnel are constantly moving in and out of corridors as they seek their destination. The vast majority of hospitals, surgery centers, and other medical facilities do not strictly regulate or closely monitor this flow of human traffic. In addition, most large medical institutions have some form of construction going on at any given period of time. Hence, it is very easy for individuals to pose as workers, visitors, students—or, even, the deli delivery guy—if such deceit is desired. A very few facilities have considered the importance of monitoring and tracking all visitors and personnel who step foot on their medical campus. For example, a company called Cemer, based in Kansas City, has created a system that uses radio frequency-activated devices to keep tabs on everyone who is present on the premises; if someone ventures to a location where he ought not to be, guards can be notified to investigate the situation.[16] This type of technical, financial (and organizational) security commitment requires a global rethinking of how an institution is run. It requires a crucial decision to treat a medical facility like any other major public landmark, which could be the site of a criminal and/or terrorist-type attack at any time.

The concept of vulnerability to violence on medical campuses is not new. During the month of January 2006, the University of Minnesota Medical Center Riverside campus was shaken when a new mother was raped. She was staying at the facility while her one-month old received treatment in the neonatal intensive care unit; the perpetrator, Abdulhai Ahmed Mohamed, was arrested and jailed shortly after the crime was revealed.[17] On September 1, 2006, in Dunn, North Carolina, Betsy Johnson Regional Hospital was notified by local police that threats had been made against the hospital. The threats were evidently motivated by the recent shooting of a black teen by police officers. Unspecified measures to beef up hospital security were reported to have been made in response to the threats. A few days earlier, in August 2006, in Virginia, a hospital security officer was shot and killed inside Montgomery Regional Hospital. In July 2006, at Howard County General Hospital in Howard County, Maryland, a fight broke out at midnight in the emergency room that left three people injured. In addition, amongst the commotion of the brawl, a suspect who was awaiting drug charges escaped custody and surveillance. In an ideal scenario, sophisticated surveillance equipment would be pared with staff who are able to indeed provide constant monitoring and provide the ability to "lock down" any given hospital department. This would require extensive training for guards, but most hospitals have only a few armed guards (if any), and little ability to successfully quarantine a trouble spot. At the Howard County General Hospital, security officers did not carry any type of weapons; only a few supervising guards even carried pepper spray.[18, 19, 20]

What the Experts Are Saying Is Very Little[21, 22]

The primary reason that hospitals and other medical facilities in America are largely unprepared to prevent and/or deal appropriately with a terrorist attack is that we have not decided to accept our vulnerability in this sector of society. In all aspects of terrorism prevention, we must learn to think like terrorists and begin to think the unthinkable. In the same vein, health care workers in Europe have begun to explore the possibilities that "terror" could unleash in a hospital setting. Authors Charles Hancock and Chris Johnson, from the University of Glasgow, devised a fictional scenario to better appreciate how bad things could get in the event of a terrorist attack against the National Health Service. In addition, they used computer simulation to more realistically understand how various facilities would confront an assault and deal with the evacuation and treatment of patients. Through these analyses, it was estimated that it would take almost six times longer to remove nonambulatory patients from a trouble zone than it would for those able to move out on their own accord. The authors, in their piece "Thinking the Unthinkable: the NHS and Terrorist Action," conclude that access to medical facilities is relatively unimpeded, that internal communication systems are mostly inadequate to deal with crisis situations, and that facilities maintain disaster response plans, which are routinely practiced by all staff members.

Some U.S. hospitals and medical personnel are moving in the right direction toward improved planning and coordination in the event a major catastrophe should occur. For example, the Northern Virginia Emergency Response Coalition (NVERC), comprising fourteen hospitals in Northern Virginia and representatives from public health agencies (as well as police/fire/rescue departments), was created to establish the framework for a workable, regional response team. This coalition was charged with developing a communications network called MEDCOMM (a direct connection with the District of Columbia's Hospital Mutual Aid Radio System). There is evidence that this type of local/regional alliance can lead to decreased costs, shared resources, a mutual buy-in on emergency protocols and procedures, and an improved delivery of medical care. This type of regional response team is a subset of the larger National Disaster Medical System (NDMS). The NDMS is a partnership between government and private entities; it is "fed" by the U.S. Department of Homeland Security (DHS), the Department of Defense (DOD), the Department of Veterans Administration, the Department of Health and Human Services, and the Federal Emergency Management Agency (FEMA). The NDMS serves to back up military operations in the event of overwhelming civilian casualties, and to respond independently to regional crises. The NVERC of the Washington, D.C. area is one of about one hundred NDMS groups throughout the country. These groups, composed of doctors, nurses, and ancillary medical support staff, train to respond to just about any type of disaster; unfortunately, they are too few and far between. The average NDMS team is composed of only about fifty to possibly one or two hundred dedicated and reliable professionals. Those making up the team are predominantly, if not exclusively, volunteers. Assuming these dedicated individuals forego taking care of their own families in a time of emergency, their effect will be limited in a city of several million reeling from a disaster of any significant proportion. The point here is not to minimize the incredible and necessary function of the NDMS regional teams, but to, again, reflect on the lack of attention currently paid to "prevention" instead of predominantly "preparedness." These volunteers should be commended for the arduous task they have agreed to confront.

It is important to recognize the significance of the previous point about giving "prevention" parity with "preparedness" efforts in terms of community planning and strategies to decrease the incidence of tragedies occurring within the U.S. health system. Consider those catastrophic entities for which prevention is of little value, and for which preparedness must take precedence:

- Major drought
- Earthquake
- Tornado
- Tsunami
- Severe snow and ice storms
- Flood
- Fire

These and other disaster scenarios are, for the most part, so far out of the realm of human control that they speak for themselves in terms of the need for adequate community planning and preparation in the event that tragedy strikes.

Now, consider those areas of society where prevention can, has, and *does* make a difference in disaster planning:

- Transportation-related failure or crash
- Power grid failure
- Contamination and/or sabotage of public utilities
- Communication system failure
- Terrorism or terrorist-like activity

Clearly, these areas demand intense scrutiny, study, and strategy to devise improved mechanisms to detect and prevent disasters from occurring in the first place. Health care is simply one of these areas that is integrally tied to all of the others; it is an area that has, unfortunately, received less attention than it deserves and needs.

In the *Journal of Homeland Security*, March 2003, Stungis and Schori describe a mathematical model, which they believe to be similar in principle to that "mindset" used by Al Qaeda in choosing targets and executing attacks. In their analyses, the authors look at a Florida County and presume ninety-nine potential terrorist "events." They then discussed the impact, circumstances, and potential measures, which could be utilized to prevent or thwart the terrorist action. Again, these writers turn to the concept of "thinking like the terrorists" and identified what they considered to be "soft" targets such as shopping malls, schools, and hospitals. The chosen Florida location of Charlotte County was not merely picked out of the air by Stungis and Schori. This spot, comprising about 150,000 residents, was the site where it is believed that Mohammed Atta and possibly several other members of the 9/11 hijack team stayed. In fact, Atta arranged overseas cash transfers, received care in a local hospital, and ate at restaurants in Charlotte County. The predominant industries of this county are local government functions, retail shops, and health care. The team of planners for the hypothetical model consisted of senior military personnel, physicians, public health care managers, experts in mathematics and physics, and specialists in psychology, infectious diseases, radiation oncology, and emergency medicine. The mathematical model concluded that the most likely location (i.e., most vulnerable, least well-guarded, and most "bang for the buck") for a terrorist attack would be the town shopping mall. Another expected target would be a sports stadium. The most likely mode of attack in the shopping mall would be "biological." Falling closely behind, other highly probable sites or events to fall victim to a terrorist attack would be as follows: festival (suicide bomb, vehicular bomb, chemical attack), shopping mall setting (chemical attack), hospital (chemical attack), food store (biological agent), hospital (biological agent), and so forth. At the bottom of the list of potential terrorist events was a vehicle bomb at either a hospital or shopping mall setting.[23]

In the scenario of a biological attack within a hospital setting, the researchers imagined three terrorists—armed with small hairspray-type containers of smallpox—contaminating the hospital cafeteria, salad bar during the lunch and dinner meals over a two-day period. They calculated that after nearly two weeks about 80 percent of the health care workers (and likely visitors) and 90 percent of patients would show signs of infection. They imagined that the perpetrators would heighten the effect of their terror by releasing videotape of their actions to the media to create a national panic. Their estimation is that the consumer markets would begin to take a nosedive and the U.S. economy would possibly spiral into a steep recession or depression.

A BRIEF GLIMPSE OF A NUCLEAR TERRORIST ATTACK[24] (THE NUCLEAR NIGHTMARE)

We have come a long way since World War II in understanding the nature of nuclear warfare, and appreciating the health risks that follow in its aftermath. In 1950, the State of California Office of Civil Defense, under then Governor Earl Warren, published the booklet *Survival Under Atomic Attack*.[25] Therein, the "Six Survival Secrets for Atomic Attacks" are revealed. Some of the pearls of wisdom offered to the public include the advice: "bury your face in your arms;" "wait at least one hour to give lingering radiation some chance to die down;" and "don't start rumors." The booklet also makes sure the reader knows not to be "misled by wild talk of super-super bombs." Unfortunately, life in the early twenty-first century is fraught with greater dangers, more numerous and more powerful bombs, and a global network of terrorists that did not exist sixty years ago. We do perhaps have more accurate and salient information at hand as we prepare to meet these modern threats.

In the world today, there is enough highly enriched uranium to make hundreds of thousands of Hiroshima-type atomic weapons. It is no secret that many thefts of such nuclear material occurred from Russian facilities in the aftermath of the fall of the former Soviet Union. Shortly after 9/11, Princeton University professor Frank von Hippel gave an interview to the *New York Times* during which he explained how relatively easy it was to create a massive nuclear explosion. A five to ten kiloton explosion (equivalent to five to ten thousand tons of TNT) can be created by dropping an approximately forty-five kilogram piece of enriched uranium 1.8 meters onto a second, similarly sized piece of enriched uranium.

In the past few years, our government has spent hundreds of millions of dollars studying and planning strategies for dealing with an urban nuclear blast—and for good reason. After such an explosion in downtown San Diego, for example—one presumably plotted to kill innocent life and take out one of the world's largest naval bases—there would be an immediate electromagnetic pulse that would knock out all electronic devices within a radius of four kilometers. The shock wave to follow would eliminate every above-ground, topographical structure and kill every living creature within a half-kilometer radius. The next half-kilometer radial band from ground zero would, likewise, be almost completely decimated. Detonation temperatures would reach millions of degrees, would ignite firestorms, and would create winds in excess of six hundred kilometers per hour. Within a few seconds, at least several hundred thousand San Diegans will have died.

In 2004, the U.S. government studied radiation injuries following a nuclear blast in an American mid-sized city. Of those not killed immediately, about 45,000 additional people would soon die, regardless of *any* subsequent medical treatment. Another roughly 250,000 people would die if denied rapid and sustained hospital treatment; and an approximate additional 150,000 individuals would require medical observation.

Radiation Sickness and the Walking Dead[26]

Accidents like the Soviet Chernobyl incident, small-scale animal studies, and military medical records of surviving Japanese following the Hiroshima and Nagasaki detonations (following World War II) provide data used by the scientific community to study radiation sickness. The smallest level of radiation exposure to animal life is termed the "gray" (one gray unit is equal to the number of joules of radiation energy absorbed per kilogram of tissue).

Radiation to humans at the level of 2–3 grays is cruelly deceptive and usually deadly. People with this level of exposure get sick, and then get better again. This latency period ultimately gives way (days to weeks) to progressive clinical symptoms, followed by death. With an incremental increase in radiation exposure, affected individuals will experience a more immediate onset of symptoms and a shorter latency phase.

The most susceptible vital organ tissue in the human body is the bone marrow (specifically, the stem cells). Stem cells are affected at the level of one-half gray unit, and are completely wiped out at about the level of five grays. Platelet and neutrophil levels begin to fall immediately, with measured levels reaching zero within days to weeks of exposure. Victims often succumb to infections and bleeding, with inherent vulnerabilities exacerbated by poor sanitation and secondary wounds associated with such a regional catastrophe. Radiation exposure exceeding five grays often leads to massive gastrointestinal tract damage—specifically to mucosal cells responsible for maintaining a safety barrier between gut bacteria and the bloodstream. The insult to these cells usually leads to massive bacteremia, septic shock, and death. The central nervous system is significantly impaired at levels of exposure nearing ten gray units.

After a nuclear disaster to any urban area (even in the best-case, homeland security response scenario), the resources to deliver palliative care to the "walking dead" will be severely limited. Under ideal recovery conditions, the key ingredients of care must consist of intravenous fluids, antimicrobial and antibiotic treatments, antiemetic agents, nutritional support, and blood transfusions.

The Bioshield Act, signed into law by the President in 2004, committed $5.6 billion to advance research (and devise better disaster response mechanisms) for dealing with chemical, biological, and nuclear agents of mass destruction. One potential new agent, G-CSF (granulocyte colony stimulating factor) is being developed by Amgen of Thousand Oaks, California. G-CSF prevents the loss of bone marrow precursor cells and contributes to the proliferation of such cells. Despite presently lacking FDA approval, Amgen has already sold large quantities of this substance to the U.S. government based on animal and human trials that have demonstrated efficacy. There remain, however, serious drawbacks to G-CSF, including a cost exceeding five thousand dollars per patient per two-week treatment period. In addition, G-CSF has an array of clinical side effects, and must remain refrigerated during storage. Lastly, G-CSF has limited effectiveness if treatment is delayed beyond several days post-exposure.

LA JOLLA, CALIFORNIA COMPANY[27]

Hollis-Eden pharmaceuticals of La Jolla has developed an inexpensive, chemically stable steroid with very few side effects. Called 5-AED (5-Androstenediol), this drug was developed as an adjunct treatment for chemotherapy patients, and was identified by government investigators as early as 1996 for the treatment of radiation injury. In trials involving rhesus monkeys, 5-AED has alleviated radiation-induced tissue damage, decreased clinical signs and symptoms of injury, and increased blood cell production. Again, this compound must be administered shortly after exposure to be effective.

SUCCESS AND FAILURE WITHIN THE U.S. BIODEFENSE INDUSTRY

Project Bioshield was created by the Federal government in 2004 to incentivize research companies to develop effective drugs and vaccines against smallpox, bubonic plague, anthrax, botulism, and other deadly agents.[28] Despite their multibillion-dollar budget, this program has yet to yield any known substantive results. The project's largest contract went to the company VaxGen Inc. in California (a total of $877.5 million) and was for the production of seventy-five-million doses of anthrax vaccine; this contract was cancelled in December 2006 because VaxGen did not meet the quality, effectiveness, and production targets set by the Department of Health and Human Services.[29]

In December 2006, President Bush signed into being the Pandemic and All-Hazards Preparedness Act and created the new Biodefense Advanced Research and Development Authority (BARDA) under the auspices of the U.S. Department of Health and Human Services.[30] The legislation for BARDA was introduced in October 2005 by the U.S. Senator of North Carolina, Richard Burr, to address the potential threats of bioterrorism. With its multiple university systems, and several well-regarded corporate research parks, North Carolina is home to the third-largest biotechnology industry in the United States. Biodefense Advanced Research and Development Authority was charged with overseeing approximately one billion dollars in funds to achieve its goals through partnerships with companies working on bioterror drugs and vaccines. There is hope that BARDA will have better success than its predecessor, Project Bioshield, but there is no way of knowing. According to many in the biotechnology industry, one of the persistent problems is that of funding and oversight. The development process is removed by BARDA from under the umbrella of the U.S. Department of Homeland Security, and is placed squarely within the U.S. Department of Health and Human Services. This is widely seen as a good thing. Nevertheless, the government has demonstrated an inadequate record in appropriating funds for these types of large projects; many companies in the past were contracted to receive payment only for the delivery of effective products—thereby creating a formidable uphill challenge for the drug industry to self-fund their own research and production.[31]

THE ROLE OF PUBLIC HEALTH AND GOVERNMENT[32]

The U.S. national government and many individual states have come up with various versions of "counterterrorism planning, planning and preparedness response" acts. These legislative actions are, arguably, necessary first steps toward better protection for our country's citizens. All of these documents contain measures to identify, study, and shore up antiterrorist measures for hospitals and other medical facilities. Nevertheless, these wordy provisions still miss the point entirely. The next wave of terrorist attacks on American soil will be devastating, regardless of whether or not they involve chemical, biological, or nuclear materials. No regional counterterrorism task force or urban search and rescue team will ever prevent an attack from occurring in the first place.

Countless articles and medical policy forums seem unable to break away from the strict "see it, isolate it, and treat it" mentality that plagues the health care political establishment across this nation. There is no doubt that physician pay, nursing satisfaction, and hazardous material treatment units are important issues, but these concerns will pale in the aftermath of a major terrorist strike against a civilian, health care establishment such as a hospital. Officials are frequently wringing their hands about the inefficient management of recent anthrax scares and the disastrous consequences of a smallpox or pneumonic plague outbreak, but fail to sense the inadequacy of basic security mechanisms presently in place in most American medical institutions. If a series of hospitals are "hit," either at one time or in random succession over time, the panic and mayhem—and psychological unrest—that will result will be immense. In the event of an attack on a hospital target, no amount of coordination between police, firefighters, paramedics, the National Guard, and mobile HAZMAT teams will be enough to quell the national anxiety that will result. The effect will be paralysis; there will be no room for regret. In April 2004, Senator Joseph Lieberman and others began to openly express their concerns that the President's Homeland Security budget was woefully incomplete and underfunded. But even Lieberman and his well-intentioned colleagues have been operating under misguided, albeit well-intentioned goals. The past few years have seen many Congressional bills and mandates such as the SAFER Act (Staffing for Adequate Fire and Emergency Response), which authorizes the U.S. Fire Administration to hire additional firefighters amongst other things. There are many other bills intended to improve bioterrorism preparedness and treatment. Nothing, however, is known to exist on the docket of any court, or the agenda of either body of Congress, to force a critical examination of the very nature of our medical system infrastructure. What this nation needs is a detailed security assessment of our acutely vulnerable facilities where the sick and infirmed are treated.

As the next two chapters will reveal, our medical institutions have weaknesses that can easily be exploited by those seeking to do us harm. In determining the threats to our hospitals, surgery centers, clinics, and medical offices, we must focus on the following general areas: the safety and security of critical equipment, arson/sabotage/theft risks, gaps in effective communication mechanisms, level and type of internal and perimeter security, drug transport, inventory and storage, patient treatment protocols, and individual patient monitoring guidelines. We must look at how our medical campuses are designed and be willing to make changes where necessary. We must examine how people enter and exit our hospitals and other medical locations. We must see (and understand) what, if anything, is done with the data collected and monitored by facility security personnel. We must consider whether our systems of personal identification merely look professional or whether they result in a tangible benefit "on the ground." In the end, we must be willing to fund upgrades in technology (cameras, motions sensors, RFID tags, etc.) that can make us truly safer.

Chance, Careless, or Criminal?

The number of American deaths due to a medical intervention over the past ten years is estimated to be 7.8 million. Almost half of these deaths are classified vaguely as "unknown cause," "medication," or "treatment"-related. This figure exceeds the number of U.S. citizens who have died in war since the nation began.[33]

6

HOSPITAL AND SURGERY CENTER "SECURITY," PART II: BREAKING IN FROM THE OUTSIDE

History is the unrolled scroll of prophecy.

—James Garfield

...We were going to operate on this prisoner. So, right before the anesthesiologist was able to place his intravenous (IV) line, the patient bolts off the table, pushes down the nurse and starts running down the hallway. The anesthesiologist grabbed a syringe of muscle relaxant and ran after him, accompanied by me. We were all afraid that the patient might hurt someone. The two of us caught up with him—like in some scene from a movie. We stabbed him in his shoulder with the medicine...it took a longer time than we'd have liked, but it did start working...this huge guy started to stumble and then just collapsed on the floor. It took five of us to hoist him up onto a gurney so we could whisk him back to the O.R. Boy, that was some strong stuff we gave him—I'd hate for it to get into the wrong hands!"

—Military surgeon

If history is already written, then it is—at best—certainly not altogether immutable. We know that our endeavors on this earth can amount to good, and that our efforts can improve the quality of life and conditions in which we live. If a man can, indeed, see the future, his best prediction would be that we seldom do enough to prevent history from repeating itself. Such could be said for our state of counterterrorism measures as they apply to the infrastructure of health care in America today.

Building on the examples of terrorism and terrorist-like attacks that have occurred to date on civilian targets in America and abroad, and upon our knowledge of the vulnerabilities inherent to medical institutions, we would do well to think like terrorists...just how would a terrorist "break in" to a hospital or other medical institution from the outside? Gaining access to the largely helpless population of patients, workers, and visitors in a civilian setting would be the initial, necessary step toward committing a crime and causing injury, death, and mayhem. Once inside a facility, many things could happen as will be addressed in the next chapter. For now, let's entertain several scenarios, or possibilities, which all represent glaring "holes" in the insufficient safety net we call "hospital security."

THE VISITOR

It is reasonable to start with the easiest method of entry into a hospital—walking through the front door as a visitor. In most medical institutions, during normal daylight hours, there is little, if any, impediment to the normal ingress and egress of visitors, delivery personnel, workers, or family members through the front lobby. Contrary to popular perception, the few hospital guards who do stand guard are more concerned with things that leave the hospital (e.g., protecting babies from being abducted from the maternity ward) than those things and people that enter the hospital. Even for those few university medical centers that sit in the middle of ostensibly "dangerous" inner-city neighborhoods, rarely are the identities of visitors checked against a verifiable and somewhat reliable identification (ID) such as a drivers license (if this were done, there would be—at the very least—some record of who was on the premises at any given time). Instead, the way things are done is that people can come and go as they please. When people are stopped (even on most maternity wards) the only requirement is to identify who they are visiting, sign a logbook (with whatever name they choose), and receive a daily ID badge. Once on the facilities, the ID badge cannot cross-reference the visitor with a name; furthermore, once on the premises, there is no way of preventing an individual from changing exterior clothing (e.g., in a public restroom) or displaying a fake badge of another sort.

As a method of insurance against dubious "visitors" to medical settings, it is always possible to conduct simple newspaper or Internet searches of accident victims to deduce the name(s) of individuals likely to be at a given facility at a given time. For perpetrators who have any access to surgeons, internists, or other specialists in or around medical facilities, rarely does a fifteen-minute interval go by when a cell phone conversation does not identify at least one name of a hospital inpatient. In other words, we should recognize that it is easy for people to overhear, or otherwise gain, private information that can be used to create a convincing, but false, impression.

The easiest way for visitors to gain unnoticed access to hospitals is to waltz through the lobby as if the expected destination is known. In a crowded, busy facility, nothing attracts less attention than confidence. An alternative method of entry would be to enter a facility lobby and simply sit down in one of the rest areas where family members congregate waiting for word about the success of a given procedure or surgery. These groups of people are often sitting, standing, talking, and making trips to the bathroom constantly throughout any given day. Since most facilities do not track individuals (more on this later), and do not keenly analyze or monitor security footage in real time, there is no chance that a given individual would be prevented from moving beyond the lobby to wherever the final destination may be.

Many facilities have back entrances leading away from cafeterias and in-house cafes. These entrances rarely, if ever, have stationed guards and provide an embarrassingly easy way to gain access to every conceivable location within an institution.

THE "HEALTH CARE WORKER"

There is a lot that can be said of the health care worker, especially once he or she is "inside" the bowels of a medical institution, but more on that later. Let's just examine the possibilities and realities of someone who is a health care worker, and how access is gained to most facilities. Physicians, nurses, technicians, administrators, vendors, pharmaceutical and supply representatives, and any other ancillary health care workers (e.g., emergency medical technicians) gain access through a variety of entry points in medical facilities. Most facilities *do not* aggressively screen ID badges person by person; in those institutions where this is done, it is rarely performed at locations other than the front lobby or other main entrance. This still leaves many other "portals" for unwanted intruders (e.g., side doors, emergency room access points, cafeteria outdoor patio doors, and administrative offices attached to the main medical campus). Even where ID badges are purportedly screened, it is almost unheard of for badges to be closely scrutinized or for individuals to be actually stopped and questioned. This means that even the most crude "fake" badges could work quite well if worn about the waist or neckline.

Even during low volume or off-peak hours, such as during the evening or early morning, health care workers are routinely required to trespass through the emergency room, adjacent radiology labs, cafeteria or lounge entry points, and other access sites. With or without a fake badge, anyone who simply adorns a white lab jacket and twenty-dollar stethoscope, wearing scrubs or clean shirt/pants with tie (or blouse/pants or dress for females) will attract no unusual attention and will be able to move about at their will without interference. In a properly secured medical facility, all health care workers would be required to register at points of entry and exit (and present ID verification individually); all individuals on the medical campus would be tracked with either permanently (full-time staff and workers) or temporarily assigned (visitors, delivery personnel, and even patients) RFID badges. These badges would be tracked by centrally located security guards and any unusual traffic patterns or movements beyond "allowed" locations would be immediately identified and the individuals located and questioned.

DELIVERY PERSONNEL

It may seem contrary to what is seen on television or in the movies, but actually most facilities likely have fairly good control over the movement of delivery personnel. Terrorists would likely not disguise themselves as the "pizza guy" or the oxygen cylinder supply guy, unless their goal was to reach a particular destination and quickly change clothing to resemble a hospital employee or physician. The reason is that those charged with delivering supplies, food, or other medical-related item are likely to stand out and be readily noticed. These individuals are more likely to draw the question "can I help you?" or "where are you going?" and they are most likely to be seen as out of place. It would be difficult to linger for any length of time in an emergency room, operating room lounge, or hospital boiler room without drawing a lot of unwanted attention.

The one big advantage that those seeking to do harm would have under the guise of a delivery person would be the ability to bring with them whatever dubious "package" they were looking to deliver to the medical facility. This ability to bring on-site some type of chemical, biological, nuclear, or simple conventional explosive device (disguised as a medical supply item or food product) makes this type of ruse particularly dangerous. It is for this reason that medical/hospital security guards should inspect each and every item that makes its way into (or out of) the facility doors. This is also a strong argument for having metal detectors, at the very least, at entrances to these institutions. Unfortunately, this practice is rarely in place at hospitals or other major medical facilities across the United States.

The "Patient" Disguise

If one considers the most porous location in any given hospital, for example, it is likely to be the emergency room. Here, patients, staff, and guests/family members all mingle in a fluid state of disarray at all hours of the day and night. Many patients may have no apparent injury, but still present themselves for evaluation of vague complaints. As these lesser acuity patients are triaged to the bottom of the list, it is not uncommon for patients to be asked to wait for many hours. While waiting, these patients frequently walk outdoors, use the restrooms, and move about the emergency department lobby. Under this circumstance, there would be ample opportunity for the criminal mind to find a way around any security guard who may be standing guard. In fact, one could argue that access to the hospital ventilation system (for the release of airborne toxins or infectious agents) would be easily obtained from the emergency room or public bathroom. Once behind the treatment doors (either by direct access or as a patient on a gurney in a patient holding bay), the opportunity to slip out and into other regions of any hospital facility would be fairly easy.

The emergency room is particularly vulnerable to any large-scale assault by multiple individuals if such an attack were desired. This is because of the way that the driveways, automatic doors, and personnel are oriented to facilitate ambulance access. Ambulances pull up and park to deliver sick patients in a fashion that is easy and unobstructed. From an ideal security standpoint, even ambulances would require some degree of automatic/electronic access to gain access to the "inner sanctuary" of the emergency department delivery area. This, however, is usually not the case; hence, terrorists seeking to deliver large payloads could do so easily at the vast majority of hospitals simply by commandeering an ambulance and knowing how to drive. This represents another glaring—yet easily fixable—loophole in how hospitals have failed to institute even the most basic of military-style "perimeters" in the aftermath of 9/11. There should be no excuse for this deficiency in security protocol. This weakness in hospital security is easily remedied.

The emergency room is also the only location in a medical facility where a patient's identification (or lack thereof), insurance verification (or lack thereof), or ability to pay, have no bearing on access to the facility. In other words, anonymity in an emergency room setting is simply not a problem. Hence, the need to create a false façade is simply one less bit of work necessary for the terrorist if he should choose to utilize this port of entry to a hospital setting.

THE FOOD SERVICE DEPARTMENT

In light of previous examples in this book demonstrating the vulnerability of cafeteria food (e.g., salad bar) to contamination with dangerous chemicals or infectious agents, one would think that such a public venue would generate a high degree of care in directly watching and/or electronically monitoring this area. Again, this is absolutely *just not done*! Medical facility food service locations tend to be high-volume departments; many are outsourced to private vendors. All are open to exploitation in the easiest of fashions. A liquid or powdery substance released from under a cuff, for example, would not be noticed in the act of reaching to obtain food from a salad bar. And, there are other ways to deliver tainted food products (or other agents—e.g., a bomb) to such a destination. The delivery docks of hospitals are large, open areas where supply trucks stop to unload their cargo. There is ample and free ingress and egress of materials that flow in and out of these locations in most medical facilities.

MEDICAL WASTE/PATHOLOGY/MORGUE

Every large medical facility or hospital contains a location for medical waste, pathology products, and dead bodies. This site usually sits within the very inner core (or lower level of the institution). Perhaps without much sophistication, and with a minimum knowledge of protocol and procedure, these areas could be easily accessed. For those seeking to gain access to other sensitive areas (central heating, ventilation systems, power plant, etc.), this would be a good place to start. Unfortunately, again, these sites contain little to no defense against unwanted entry or nefarious schemes.

Playing the odds, and considering the terrorist's goal of seeking to coordinate and implement large-scale fear, panic, and death, it is likely that they would utilize the hospital/medical setting to implement a more subtle form of attack. Why blow up a hospital, when you can poison IV fluid bags, ventilation systems, or salad bars at multiple locations, and then later take credit for the unfolding mayhem? Why kill ten people in a brazen emergency room attack, when you can use the institution's own internal mechanisms to carry out the killing of hundreds of people in a way that is not easily detected. One of the major accomplishments of the 9/11 terrorists was the ability to inflict billions of dollars of expense, hardship (and time) to the daily lives and routines of all Americans. If simple, upgraded security measures are not put into place now to better secure America's hospitals, surgery centers, and other medical facilities, then we the taxpayers will be mourning unnecessary deaths and writing even larger checks to fortify these institutions in the aftermath of the next attack. Despite measures by the Federal government to minimize public concern over such matters, we know that our elected officials have largely opted to hope for a pass by our enemies in this aspect of homeland security, in lieu of actually shoring up our defenses. What a shame it would be if every American citizen, every loved one, and every patient were to have to carry with him the same degree of underlying—if not unspoken—fear he now shuttles aboard an airplane. As a society, we can do a better job of securing our health care institutions.

THEY CHEERED ON 9/11 (A BRIEF COMMENTARY AND PERSONAL STORY)

This story was incorporated into a "letter to the editor" to several U.S. magazines and newspapers, including the New York Times and the San Jose Mercury News (in response to articles they had run about 9/11). The letters were rejected for publication—no reasons were given.

Back in the Summer/Fall of 2001, this author was the new chief of anesthesiology of an ailing inner-city hospital on the East Coast. I had decided to take the job partly because it was near where I had completed my residency training a decade earlier; and it was my hope to draw upon local contacts to elevate the lesser-known hospital's quality of medicine. As it turned out, it was to be an unachievable challenge.

Within weeks of taking over the reigns of that department, it was discovered that internal stealing by the office manager had been going on for years; in addition, several nonboarded anesthesiologists were revealed to have had less than stellar clinical records. Further investigation brought forth evidence that the hospital had been engaged in irregular billing practices for a decade (the Federal government was eventually brought in to look into allegations of Medicare and Medicaid fraud). My personal efforts to improve the quality of medicine made small gains, but were mostly met with resistance. Because a sizable percentage of the hospital's medical staff was not board-certified in their specialty, they feared any sweeping movement for change that could threaten their positions. The hospital eventually agreed to dismiss the office manager, but its vice president (VP) for medical affairs refused to push for legal redress against the former employee because it would (his words, private conversation) "reflect poorly on me, the vice president."

In what would prove to be a five-year mission, fraught with local political pressure (intended, it appeared, to protect the reputation of the larger health system that owned the hospital), the Medicare fraud lawsuit against that hospital—*and on behalf of the U.S. Government*—was settled. The CEO had been forced to resign, and the hospital admitted wrongdoing in its settlement in 2005. I quickly sought an exit strategy from that flawed institution, and left eighteen months after starting. I consider my efforts successful, at least, in helping to put an end to health insurance fraud. Interestingly, only months after my departure, an employee in that same hospital's laboratory made national headlines by exposing evidence that multiple patients had been given the wrong result for their HIV tests. This astute lab technician's actions prompted an overhaul in that state (and nationwide) of how clinical laboratories are evaluated and accredited.

Looking back on that hospital experience, I remember a day that is now seared in my memory—the day we were attacked by Al Qaeda. On September 11, 2001, on that hospital's seventh floor, in a grungy staff lounge, several Middle-Eastern physicians stood around the lone television and cheered. I had been in the operating room, but was quickly informed about the series of attacks on American soil that were unfolding. The cheering doctors, who happened to be foreign-trained surgeons from Islamic countries, were commenting: "the U.S. is getting what they deserve . . . let's see what these Jew-lovers have to say now." My heart sank; I felt sicker than any patient I had ever seen recovering from anesthesia. The horror and loss of innocent life, coupled with a sense of fear from terrorist sympathizers who were standing just a few feet away, was unbearable. I wanted to get away, but I couldn't; I had to return to the operating room for more cases. I wanted to go home, grab my family, and run for safety, but I was trapped at work with people who hated me and wanted my country destroyed.

Those doctors, who jumped for joy upon seeing the carnage of the Twin Towers in New York, and the attack on the Pentagon, are still among us. To them, the glory of our open, democratic society is not seen as a national treasure, but merely an opportunity to undermine our national security. They are not seeking to graciously assimilate and contribute to American culture, but rather to stand apart and secretly plot against it. The terrorist sympathizers are just as dangerous as the terrorists themselves—they sap our resources and wait for an opportune moment when we are vulnerable.

Today, more that ever before in our country's history, we must resolve to look beyond our political parties and jointly face the foe of radical Islam. This is not a slur against Muslims or a particular nationality (however, peace-loving Muslims have made themselves irrelevant by their own silence). It is a stark picture of the intentions of the fundamentalist Islamist movement. These individuals seek to infiltrate and overthrow our way of life—killing whoever stands in their way. Our nation's next major foreign policy priority might be the Islamic Republic of Iran, whose radical clerics would like to ignite a nuclear holocaust against Israeli, European, and American targets if given the chance.

We cannot make the mistake that Chamberlain made before World War II, and we cannot afford to underestimate the evils evident in today's world.

Nearly three thousand U.S. citizens were slaughtered on 9/11. On that fateful day, foreign doctors stood on American soil—with work visas and an opportunity for a better life in hand—and rejoiced at our suffering.

HOW A MEDICAL DRUG WAS FATALLY EMPLOYED AGAINST TERRORISTS[1, 2]

Over eight hundred moviegoers were taken hostage in a Moscow theater on October 23, 2002. The perpetrators, all forty-one of them, were Chechen separatists who identified their group as the "Islamist Suicide Squad" (ISS). At around 9 p.m., the attack began, setting into motion a crisis that would last until the early morning hours of October 27, 2002. Some of the terrorists were wearing powerful explosive belts, designed to ward off a precipitous raid by the Russian Special Forces. The Chechens also carried with them machine guns, various small arms, and ammunition. The ISS demanded an end to the war in Chechnya and full Chechen independence. They declared that hostages would be shot, starting at the twelfth hour; the Russian authorities never established any serious negotiating effort. The crisis ended when the Russian Special Forces pumped an aerosolized version of the narcotic fentanyl (one hundred times more potent and faster acting than morphine) into the theater's ventilation system. The gas quickly subdued the terrorists, and the Russian forces moved in. The fentanyl gas resulted in the death of both Chechens and hostages—in all, forty-one terrorists died (all of them) and 129 hostages were killed (127 of whom died as a result of fentanyl inhalation).

Fentanyl is a synthetic opioid, available by prescription only. It is an extremely potent painkiller, used predominantly for anesthesia in the IV form. It also comes in a patch form (e.g., chronic pain sufferers; cancer patients) and as a lollipop (e.g., used to sedate children before the induction of anesthesia). Prior to October 27, 2002, the gaseous form of fentanyl had never been used—or even described in the scientific literature. Fentanyl is a highly addictive substance, sometimes identified on "the street" as the recreational drug called China White. Its use causes constriction of the pupils, nausea with vomiting, and a combination of drowsiness and euphoria. The drug kills through its strong effect of respiratory depression—recipients begin to take progressively more shallow breaths until they become hypoxic, unconscious, and then die. Brain cells become irreversibly damaged at approximately three minutes of oxygen deprivation (hypoxia); complete brain death occurs when low blood oxygen levels are sustained for greater than six minutes. Fentanyl, like morphine, is a chemical derivative of the drug heroin.

The Moscow theater terrorist attack is concerning on its face—hundreds of people were frightened beyond belief and brutalized; in the end, 170 of them—innocents and terrorists—were dead. This event is ominously frightening, however, for other reasons. First, it marked the new use of an established, medical-grade drug. There is no doubt that terrorists worldwide have since studied the pharmacology of applying fentanyl to their own laundry list of potential weapons. Second, the attack is troubling because of how it was planned and carried out. The Chechens literally smuggled a large cache of weapons and explosives undetected across thousands of miles to their destination in downtown Moscow. Lastly, there is no reason to believe that terrorists here in the United States could not gain access to theatres, retail outlets, hospitals, or doctors' offices (to name only a few locations) and unleash panic and disaster in ways we have previously thought impossible.

Chance, Careless, or Criminal?

A 2001–2002 survey of 7,000 American hospital executives revealed that only 5 percent placed researching the cause of unknown or preventable medical errors (and medical-related deaths) as a "top priority."[3]

7

HOSPITAL SECURITY, PART III: THINKING LIKE A TERRORIST—THE INSIDE JOB

There is no security on this Earth. Only opportunity.

—General Douglas MacArthur

...I was scared. Three gunshots had rung out—POP. POP. POP. People were screaming. I didn't know what was going on. No one talks about it, even to this day."

—Emergency room clerk

Anyone with an explosive device and the will to commit evil can and will find a way to sow destruction in just about any setting. This sentiment can just as easily be applied to health care institutions as it could to other public places; although, it is far more likely that perpetrators of crimes against medical targets will apply a degree of subtlety and "inside" knowledge if their intentions are to kill and instill a sense of profound fear because their methods are less than easily detected and thus more insidious and "unknown." After all, a bomb simply "goes off"—we sort of already know this drill! The local police, FBI, ATF, and others move in to clean up the mess, track down clues, and pursue those responsible. In general, however, the public is not so familiar with the intricacies of today's modern "tools of medicine"—especially if these "tools" are suddenly turned against us. Frankly, it is this concept that constitutes what this book is essentially all about—putting to print glaring, inherent weaknesses in our health care system that could (read: "probably will") be implemented at some point in our history if we (the educated public) do not recognize (and shore up) our vulnerabilities. This chapter will review further the government's perspective on the terrorist threat to medical institutions and some fundamental issues pertinent to internal hospital security; we will then move on to detail several scenarios of potential "attack" that could easily occur in most hospitals or surgery centers in the United States today. These scenarios build on information, criminal case history, and methods already developed thus far in this book.

THE GOVERNMENT'S PERSPECTIVE IS FOCUSED ON EMERGENCY MEDICAL RESPONSE[1]

Our government is preoccupied with those issues surrounding the Emergency Medical Response system—i.e., that system in place, on both a national and regional level, that musters resources and administers care to victims of natural disasters, crises involving mass civilian casualties, and other catastrophic events. Even today, despite what government officials would like us to believe, we remain on "defense." The reason we are incapable of moving to the next level of security is because we are preoccupied with what we can see—not with what we can imagine; we are fixated on what we "have"—not on what we *should* have in terms of proper security measures within our national health care infrastructure.

On September 11, 2001, over 3,300 people were killed and more than 10,000 people were injured in the attacks against the twin towers in New York, the Pentagon in Virginia, and the plane headed for the U.S. capital that went down in the fields of rural Pennsylvania. In the 1993 attack against the World Trade Center in New York, 6 people were killed and more than 1,000 injured. In April 1995, during the bombing of the Federal Building in Oklahoma City, 168 people were killed and hundreds others injured. In 1996, a pipe bomb was detonated in Centennial Park in Atlanta, Georgia during the Olympic games, killing 2 people and wounding 110 others. The attacks against four commuter trains in March 2004 in Madrid, Spain, resulted in the death of 190 people and the injury of over 1,800 others. Subsequent to this, Muslim radicals believed to be of Pakistani origin have killed hundreds of train passengers in India in several distinct, coordinated bombing attacks. These types of attacks represent the status quo in today's world. Although the basic infrastructure of American society has not yet been disrupted, our world has forever changed because of fundamental underlying current of unrest and fear against the next, inevitable attack. It should be inherently obvious that the terrorists are equally intelligent and clever as we; and it should be evident that the terrorists are constantly thinking of ways to exploit our open society. They have to be successful only once to celebrate and dance in the streets; we have to be successful 100 percent of the time.

In our present system of "security defense," we are relying on a complex network of civil, military, and volunteer citizen-based organizations and agencies to be cooperative in the aftermath of an attack. Aside from political and jurisdictional conflicts, this web of "first responders" and caregivers must communicate continuously to insure that resources are properly allocated. In effect, the network of firemen, local police, emergency medical technicians, Federal authorities, intelligence analysts, military units, and health care workers must clean up the mess that has already happened. In any attack of substantial magnitude (i.e., one that involves a coordinated, simultaneous assault on multiple medical facilities), the damage to our medical response system and the depletion of our marginally adequate health care resources will send our hospitals, surgery centers, and emergency medical response units into crisis mode. Even if every agency from the local fire station to the Director of the Federal Emergency Management Association (FEMA) is working at top capacity and efficiency, we will have already begun falling into "catch-up mode." Elective surgeries, treatments, and interventions will need to be placed on hold in a swath of hundreds of miles around the regional focus of attack. The national mentality of fear and uncertainty will rise and public panic will begin to take hold. The stock market will plummet and the national economy will reflect a depression in output. This spiral of havoc and chaos is preventable but only if we begin to take actions to identify and fix intra-health care security weaknesses today! The reason that hospitals and other health care facilities are such a natural target for attack is that they represent the crucial link in any disaster response plan. In the same way that the Human Immunodeficiency Virus (HIV) has confounded a successful cure by attacking the disease-fighting white blood cells themselves (causing so much misery and loss of life), terrorists will gain maximal leverage in an attack by striking at the heart of our emergency response mechanism: our treatment facilities.

Today's health care manuals and disaster treatment scenarios detail copious pages of protocols to insure that residual explosives and contaminants do not remain to confound rescue and treatment efforts. They emphasize that "safety perimeters" be established and that victims and rescue workers receive proper "decontamination" at various intervals after any given attack. There are also substantial guidelines explaining how toxic agents are neutralized, transported, and disposed of in the most effective and safe manner. These emergency standards are essential as a last resort, but absolutely cannot be acceptable alone because no amount of mobile, MASH-type treatment tents can substitute for the hospital itself. Although national and regional authorities should create a formal registry of licensed, freestanding surgical facilities to function as an emergency backup to our hospital system (ambulatory surgery centers contain functional, fully equipped operating rooms and postanesthesia care units that could replace hospital operating rooms in the event of an emergency), the best answer remains better preparation to decrease the likelihood of attack in the first place. Let us move on to examine those conventional agents of destruction that could most likely be used in an internal attack against a medical target, then look at the limited methods of security presently in place at most health care institutions.

Potential Agents of Destruction "From Within"[2–4]

We have previously touched on the more subtle ways to subvert the medical establishment against its own patients and will revisit this issue again with more examples at the end of this chapter. Meanwhile, let's begin by looking in more detail at those lethal agents already identified as hazards to any public setting.

Conventional Explosives

Since bags, purses, and briefcases are not routinely—if ever—screened by security personnel at hospital entrances, and since the use of metal detectors is a rare exception at medical facilities, conventional explosives remain a significant risk to the health care setting. These items are relatively easy to obtain, manufacture, and devise; furthermore, despite cursory methods to regulate firearms and monitor the flow of explosive materials in the United States, there is an abundance of available compounds to produce conventional bombs. The fundamental physics of an explosive device is the creation of a rapidly expanding chemical reaction that converts a solid or liquid precursor agent into an expanding gas. Although some bombs contain harmful pellets or shards of metal to increase their destructive capacity, their primary lethal mechanism stems from the creation of an exponential increase in atmospheric pressure in the immediate surrounding area. All conventional explosives rely on a fuel source, and, unfortunately, medical facilities often contain huge caches of fuel—in the form of oxygen tanks and oxygen lines run throughout most walls, floors, and ceiling spaces—to expand even the most minimal explosion into a towering inferno. The information provided here requires no sophisticated references or complex explanations—it should be painfully obvious! Striking an oxygen storage facility within a hospital is analogous to blowing up an eighteen-wheeled fuel truck sitting at a gas station at the base of an oil refinery. As oil flows upwards and outward from its source through a system of pipes and riggings, so does oxygen throughout the walls of a hospital. Unlike the oil refinery, there is usually no complex system of locked doors and gates—no central shut-off valves or security cameras—to monitor this medical facility Achilles heel. It is imperative that legislators, health care administrators and hospital architects re-examine this fundamental weakness to preclude the possibility that an unthinkable disaster scenario could even occur.

Almost instantaneously after the trigger of a conventional explosive, there is the initial "shock" called a positive pressure wave; following this is the phase where the displaced gases (air) move back in to fill the void created by the initial wave. This second stage is called the negative pressure wave. Both waves cause damage to surrounding structures and life. Conventional explosives are classified by low-grade and high-grade categories to describe the type, process, and destructive potential of the agent. Low-grade explosives occur in the form of certain types of gunpowder, commercial fireworks, simple rocket propellants, nitrocellulose, and nitrostarch. High-grade explosives, which are also used as detonation devices for nuclear bombs, are considered more chemically stable than their low-grade counterparts. Nitroglycerin is the famous predecessor to all modern high-grade explosives. Although nitroglycerin is used extensively in the operating room and intensive care units to decrease blood pressure and preserve cardiac function in severely ill patients, the quantities and concentration of medical nitroglycerin place it far below the threshold necessary for an explosive hazard. Ammonium nitrate, TNT, C-3, C-4, Amatol

80/20, PETN, RDX, Composition B, and the classic "dynamite" are other examples of high-grade explosives. To start the chain-reaction that creates a high-grade explosion, "initiators" are needed. Common initiators include lead azide and styphnate.

Since the destructive potential of a conventional explosive is created by shock waves (i.e., the expansion and contraction of the surrounding air—hence the loud sound associated with explosions), it is only logical that the more confined the space in which the blast occurs the more destruction will result. Closed spaces create reflected shock waves, which can compound and amplify the original blast wave. Similarly, the death and destruction caused by explosions that occur inside narrow hallways or tunnels (e.g., parking complexes or storage areas located at the foundation of a structure), can be exponentially increased in the same way a bullet is channeled through a rifle. When describing injuries caused by blasts, it is common to refer to first-, second-, and third-level damage. The primary injury is caused by the tremendous change in pressure caused at the inception of the explosion. From an anatomic and physiological perspective, the primary blast will create damage to the ears, nervous system, lungs, and often the cardiovascular system as well. Occasionally, the intestinal system is likewise affected. Common clinical conditions seen with the primary explosion include abnormal blood and air inside the lung cavity (hemothoraces and pneumothoraces), blunt injury of the heart muscle and blood inside the cardiac sac (cardiac contusion), rupture of the esophagus, perforation of the bowel and other digestive organs, and pockets of air that are forced into the vascular system and act like clots to stop circulation (arterial gas embolism).

Secondary blast injuries result when metal, glass, wood, plastic, rubber, stone, and other particles become projectiles and lodge in areas of the body. As an example, the 1996 Atlanta Olympic Games bomber used screws, nuts, and other metal shards as projectiles to heighten the extent of injury from his improvised explosive device. In addition to direct human injury, the secondary blast injuries can be exacerbated if these flying particles impale oxygen or other flammable containers or pipes, thus resulting in a cascade of mayhem. The classification of tertiary or third-level injury includes those myriad of bodily damage that occurs when people themselves are thrown large distances from the initial force of the blast.

Chemicals and Toxic Compounds[5]

In 1969, the United Nations defined chemical warfare agents as chemicals in any form that are used to kill animals or plant life. Considering that well over 100,000 relatively common industrial compounds are considered toxic, the potential for chemicals to be misused is high. Chemical agents were first used on a large scale to kill during World War I. Although toxic chemical agents are easier to obtain and/or synthesize than biological or nuclear weapons, their use against civilians in the setting of a medical building or hospital would likely be limited to an airborne route and have lower numbers of overall casualties. Chemicals may be spread by airflow and water, but are also limited by the principle of dilution and adherence. As toxins become less concentrated and bind to environmental structures, they become less available to kill living creatures. Experts divide chemical warfare agents into two categories: lethal and nonlethal. Nonlethal agents include those that weaken the neuromuscular system and cause some form of incapacitation, as well as those that cause other systemic irritations such as vomiting or excessive tearing. Lethal agents include toxic nerve agents, airway-constricting agents, and cyanides (which rapidly shut down cellular metabolism and cause almost immediate death). It is worth going through the types of chemical agents specifically, because it allows an opportunity to reflect on how these compounds could be planted in various central locations of a facility's ventilation system, or left in areas of high personnel density (e.g., lobby, operating room, and emergency room). It is theoretically possible that terrorists could infiltrate central locations where water comes into facilities, and thus contaminate the supply line; having said this, it is extremely unlikely that this route of attack would be utilized. Contaminating water would require such vast quantities of agent as to preclude any significant consequences. Furthermore, in order to instill large-scale panic and disruption, terrorists would want to attack multiple facilities simultaneously or lead the public to believe that future attacks of this type are likely. Terrorists would most likely utilize some form of airborne route, especially considering the relative ease with which individuals can move around freely on medical campuses.

Tear Gas

Perhaps the most famous of the nonlethal chemical agents is tear gas. Tear gas is considered a lacrimator—i.e., a chemical substance that induces an incapacitating degree of upper respiratory drainage, eye irritation, burning and discharge, light sensitivity, and some degree of breathing difficulty. Utilized as a law enforcement and military tool, the expected effect of these agents is not death; in fact, a full and rapid recovery can be obtained by changing clothes and washing with soap and water. Examples of "tear gas" include: chloroacetophenone and chloropicrin (in chloroform), chloroacetophenone (in chloroform), bromobenzyl cyanide, orthochlorobenzylidenemalonitrile, dibenzoxazepine, and 2-chloroacetophenone. It is unlikely that terrorists would bother with this type of agent as it does not satisfy their desire for death and destruction.

Nausea Gases

"Nausea gases" or emesis-inducing agents are respiratory and skin irritants that result in severe nausea and vomiting. These chemicals include diphenylcyanoarsine, diphenylchloroarsine, and adamsite. Again, washing the body and clothing effectively neutralizes this type of agent. The other common nonlethal type of chemical agent is that category which includes incapacitating agents such as mescaline, psilocybin, psilocin, and lysergic acid diethylamide (LSD). The military has experimented with the use of the compound benzilate, which causes dizziness, vomiting, blurred vision, confusion, and rapid heart rate for several hours after exposure. This agent is not absorbed via the skin, but does gain entry to the body through mucous membranes (e.g., mouth and nose) and attacks the respiratory system. Death is not a common or expected outcome after exposure to "nausea gas" chemicals.

Cyanide Compounds

This category of lethal chemical agents includes cyanide compounds, vesicants, nerve agents, and choking agents. These agents can be lethal by any means that introduces them to the body's circulatory system and cellular processes—usually by ingestion, mucous membrane contact, or inhalation. These agents are inherently deadly, and hence are more difficult to handle and distribute without causing death in the perpetrator. They remain viable options for terrorists, however, because small containers could be rigged with timers to conceal and later release the agent at central locations within a closed space (or for uptake by a facility's ventilation system).

Cyanide compounds, such as hydrogen cyanide and cyanogen chloride, have been used in warfare since World War I. Unless treated almost immediately, cyanide poisoning causes a rapid and irreversible death by putting a cog in the wheel of cellular respiration (the cyclical process of "cellular breathing" that transforms ATP—adenosine triphosphate—into AMP—adenosine monophosphate). Poisoning with a cyanide compound produces outward signs of seizures, paralysis of the breathing mechanism, coma, and death. Theoretically, cyanide poisoning can be treated with a combination of nitrites and thiosulfates, both of which are available in commercial kits for the military. In reality, no one survives poisoning with cyanide—it simply *doesn't happen* unless the dosage of poison is extremely diluted, and sophisticated medical help is immediately available! Cyanide and cyanide derivatives are the type of chemical compounds that could realistically be employed against helpless civilians within a hospital or other medical facility. The near-absolute success in rendering victims dead (at low cost)—and their ability to be produced in private laboratories—make cyanide compounds a likely choice of poison by terrorists.

Blistering Agents

The common term for chemical vesicants is "blistering agent." These compounds—the best known of which is Mustard Gas (also originally used in World War I)—cause blisters and irritation to the skin, eyes, and respiratory system. Blistering agents also cause gastrointestinal irritation and result in bloody sputum, shortness of breath, painful lesions, and peeling of the skin. In addition to intense pain, these agents eventually result in shock (from the loss of fluids and blood, and the inability to properly regulate body temperature) and death. Although symptoms may not immediately appear after exposure, any significant contact with chemical vesicants will lead to an irreversible process for which there is no antidote. Other kinds of blistering agents include lewisite (which results in immediate symptoms), sulfur mustard, phosgene oxime, nitrogen mustard, and agent T.

Nerve Agents

The category of chemicals known as "Nerve Agents" are basically derivatives of common insecticides, and chemically similar to drugs used in the operating room, intensive care unit, and emergency room on a routine basis. Nerve agents block the normal process by which chemical signals travel from one nerve ending to the next; the medical term is called acetylcholinesterase inhibitors. In other words, these agents paralyze their victims—whether insect, animal, or human. The result is an inability to breath, a deprivation of oxygen (hypoxia), and then brain death followed by internal organ failure. Initially, victims may salivate (because they are unable to swallow their oral secretions); urination, defecation, and even vomiting can be seen in victims of nerve agent attack. Although the effects of a nerve agent attack could result in death by a simple droplet making contact with the skin, this route of contamination is much less likely to result in injury than if the substance is inhaled (or has contact with the mucous membranes of the mouth or eyes). Mucous membranes allow rapid absorption of drugs, infectious agents, and chemicals into the bloodstream. Antidote drugs such as atropine sulfate, if injected in high doses, can reverse the (autonomic nervous system) side effects of nerve agents; atropine works by countering the low heart rate and excessive salivation that result from the nerve agents. Only direct competitors for the neuromuscular endplate (such as pralidoxime, pyridostigmine, and neostigmine) can reverse the paralysis caused by nerve agents, and potentially save a victim from death. In some cases, intended victims can be injected with these "reversal agents" before an attack to offer some degree of protection. This pretreatment only works if the half-life of the antidote drug remains in the bloodstream longer than the chemical poison.

Examples of other nerve agents include Sarin, Soman, VX Gas, and Tabun. VX Gas is considered the most dangerous of the nerve agents because it remains extremely stable once it has bound to body tissues; it also demonstrates very little volatility, and thus is less likely to evaporate or wash away. The ultimate and most reliable treatment for nerve agent attack is the placement of an artificial airway (most reliably an endotracheal tube between the vocal cords) to breath for the victim; the placement of cardiac monitors and an intravenous (IV) line (to identify and treat aberrations in cardiopulmonary function) will also be necessary. Regardless of whether victims of nerve agent attack have received antidote treatment or not, they should be immediately triaged to a mobile treatment tent, emergency room, or operating room for management by an anesthesiologist, nurse anesthetist, and/or emergency medical specialist.

Chlorinated Compounds

Chlorinated compounds, which are relatively easy to obtain, can be used as choking agents. Once exposed to the respiratory tract by inhalation, chlorine gas can cause shortness of breath, chest tightness and burning, and eventually cessation of breathing and death. Chlorine works by inducing a profound irritation of the delicate lining of the respiratory system, causing tissues to swell and ultimately occlude the breathing tubes. The small air sacs of the lung, alveoli, fill up with a foamy, bloody, cellular fluid in a condition known as pulmonary edema. Although the chlorine can be neutralized with inhaled, nebulized sodium bicarbonate, the mainstay of treatment consists of maintaining a patent airway, giving oxygen, administering IV glucocorticord steroids (to treat inflammation), and starting a course of diuretics to allow the body to absorb and clear away excess fluid in the lungs. Occasionally, placement of a breathing tube is necessary for adequate oxygenation and to allow deep suction of the lungs to clear away excess fluid.

Biological Weapons[5]

In 1972, the United States, along with sixty-nine other nations signed The Biological and Toxin Weapons Convention. This document banned the use of weaponized biological agents. No one can claim with certainty that biological agents have been used in any large-scale fashion during wartime. Nevertheless, we are all aware of attempts to use anthrax (or a substitute, "fake" white powder) to kill and produce mass hysteria—examples of which have already been introduced in this book. Biological agents hold a dark promise for terrorists because they have the potential to create illness and death on a scale that can potentially even exceed that of nuclear weapons. Once a biological agent has taken hold in a population, the possibility of spread from one individual to the next can extend the effectiveness of this "weapon" and deplete millions upon millions (if not billions) of dollars in resources, hours of lost work, etc. from a given population. Thus, biological weapons have the potential to be profoundly effective; they are, however, tricky to "grow," sustain, and deliver.

Thinking like a terrorist can sometimes be confounding, but in the case of biological agents we can be fairly sure of some things. First, terrorists will likely not make their intentions immediately clear, allowing them to evade capture (and their cause to capitalize on the incubation interval to plan further attacks between delivery and evidence of a local epidemic). The origin of the infectious entity will soon become evident to authorities. Furthermore, the perpetrators will more than likely prefer to infect multiple different geographic locations within a given region so that it will be apparent that the source of infection was deliberate and with malice. Unlike the brainwashed, generally uneducated "suicide bombers" of the Middle East, those who seek out North American targets for attack—be they domestic or foreign—will be more sophisticated if their goal is to disseminate biological agents. They will probably be less interested in dying for their cause if that death is meant to be slow and agonizing over the course of days to weeks. They will likely be too valuable to act carelessly, or with disregard for the nature of their weapon. Those terrorists using biological weapons will want to strike again and again, applying their knowledge, training, and stockpile of agents to multiple locations as they try to elude law enforcement.

Predicting the More Likely Biological Weapon

Anthrax (B. Anthracis)

Some biological agents have already been introduced in this text, but here we shall refrain from merely listing agents. Instead, we will postulate as to which ones are more likely to be used as weapons against civilian targets. Predicting agents of death is not a pleasant task, but necessary if we are to successfully prepare for the next attack on our soil. Americans are already familiar with anthrax (Bacillus anthracis), a bacteria that causes destruction of tissues and bleeding primarily in the lungs and chest cavity. Death can occur within two to three days, although life-supporting mechanisms can sustain individuals for longer before they ultimately succumb. Unless antibiotics are given very early in the course of an infection, even the strongest antibacterial drugs given IV usually cannot reverse the progressive destruction of normal organs that leads to death. A vaccine is now available, and the oral antibiotics doxycycline and ciprofloxacin can be effective against anthrax if given early enough. Emergent Biosolutions produces the only FDA-approved vaccine for the prevention of anthrax disease.[6] The vaccine is called BioThrax, and is not known to be effective after the exposure to anthrax has occurred. The vaccine cannot be used in children or pregnant women.

The following are other biological agents likely to be used in a biological attack:

Brucellosis (Brucella Species)

Brucellosis is extremely contagious and infectious, but more responsive than anthrax to treatment; it is thus less lethal. The most common cause of death from infections with the Brucella species is endocarditis; other common morbidities include infections of the gastrointestinal tract and the genitourinary tract, bone infections, and a high fever. There is no FDA-approved vaccine available at this time for Brucellosis.

Smallpox (Variola Major)

Smallpox remains a potentially terrifying viral "weapon". Except for rare reports, the last significant patch of smallpox infection was reported in the late 1970s. As a result, for a long time there were no active programs for smallpox vaccination, and there existed no significant stockpiles of smallpox vaccine available to the general public. This, however, does not mean that smallpox vaccines do not presently exist in the ledgers of public inventory. Because of threat of bioterrorism resulting from new strain cultures (or those known to exist in the confines of the CDC in Atlanta, Georgia, and the Research Institute of Viral Preparations in Moscow, Russia), the United States has recently commissioned the production of vaccines for this disease. It is believed that by the end of the year 2007, there will exist in the collective U.S. stockpiles at least one vaccine per American citizen.[7] Smallpox is dangerous because it can be spread easily by means of aerosol and can create a disabling fever, delirium, rash, and pneumonia. The most common cause of death is by secondary bacterial infection of the lungs.

Ebola (Hemorrhagic Fever)

Variants of the Ebola virus can cause an extremely potent, hemorrhagic viral infection sometimes called Rift Valley fever. Symptoms can include generalized weakness, fever, dehydration, loss of vascular integrity, and impaired cardiopulmonary function. The severe risk of this class of virus is its ability to be transmitted and contracted extremely easily (via any form of direct contact) and its ability to cause high rates of mortality. Although some vaccines may be available for certain strains, an outbreak in unprotected populations can cause death rates well in excess of 50 percent. If terrorists were to get a hold of a powerful strain of this type of virus, and manage to unleash it into dense populations such as the captive audience of patients and workers in a hospital setting, the rapidly unfolding sickness and sheer number of victims would quickly overwhelm any regional health system.

Encephalitis Viruses; Miscellaneous Biological Agents

Various forms of the encephalitis viruses, including the Eastern, Western, and Venezuelan equine forms, may be quite available to terrorists seeking to obtain them. These viruses, in the absence of a vaccinated population (not all strains have vaccines), can cause progressive lethargy, seizure, weakness, and death in rates up to 75 percent.

There are other infectious diseases which could be purposefully disseminated to cause sickness and death in any given population. These can include Clostridium botulinum (most commonly causes respiratory weakness and paralysis), Coxiella burnetii (known as Q fever; most commonly causes malaise only), and Yersinia pestis (the plague).

It is alarming to note that the following (additional) deadly biologic agents either have no commercially available vaccine in the United States, or the use of a vaccine has been deemed inefficient and potentially dangerous:[8]

- Botulism (C. botulinum)
- Hemorrhagic fever viruses (Ebola and Marburg families)
- Pneumonic plague (Yersinia pestis)
- Q fever (Coxiella burnetii)
- Eastern, Western, and Venezuelan equine encephalitis (Alpha viruses)

- Typhus fever (Rickettsia prowazekii)
- Staphylococcus (Enterotoxin B)
- Hanta virus
- Nipah virus
- Melioidosis or Glanders (Burkholderia mallei, Burkholderia pseudomallei)

A Brief Mention of "Lasers"

No discussion of "weapons" or potential tools of terrorism would be complete without mentioning lasers. Although highly unlikely today, the presence of early prototypes of "directed-energy weapons" in military arsenals worldwide indicates the certainty that terrorists will someday begin using these lasers to kill. Without getting into unnecessary detail, laser weapons work by creating electromagnetic energy in a highly focused stream that travels at the speed of light. Once operational, these weapons may be less expensive and easier to use than conventional, biological, chemical, or nuclear weapons. Lasers work on a greater, more powerful scale much like the simple light pens used by lecturers attempting to point out a spot on a projection screen before a large audience. Imagine the use of a military-grade laser unit that could cause retinal damage and incapacitate large numbers of people, so as to allow the planting of another lethal device or compound within a health care setting. The blinding effect of the laser could also be used to confuse video surveillance units in an attempt to penetrate restricted areas.

HOSPITAL SECURITY (OR LACK THEREOF)

Most of what follows in this book is as real as any scientific fact referenced in this text. The primary source, however, is the author. Although many people possess the information I am offering, no one is writing about it; few care enough to lend their insights. The sad truth is that apart (perhaps, we hope) from experts working for the Department of Homeland Security and other national organizations, there is no comparable information "out there" for public consumption. Some may like to believe that our elected officials, in their wisdom and charity, have gone to great lengths to insure multiple layers of secret security for our nation's precious and acutely vulnerable medical facilities. I cannot allow myself to be deluded into such a belief. Clearly, in the powerful capitalistic engine that drives our economy, we would see far more activity by security firms and high-tech gurus trying to gain market share for the multibillion-dollar task of securing our health care sites. Thus, we are left with the task of promoting this cause from the ground up—or, as we might say, "from the bedside to the boardroom." The title of this book was chosen carefully, because the battle waged by extremists (who would like nothing better than to lay ruin to our freedoms) is moving our way. It is only a matter of time before our homeland is struck again; it is only a matter of time before American medical facilities are targeted.

We would be entertaining a fantasy to believe that most U.S. hospital security forces are routinely capable of (or actively busy) doing anything other than responding to the occasional emergency room scuffle, the parking lot break-in, or the goodwill service of shuttling employees to their vehicles at the end of late-night shifts. It would be folly to assume that security firms hired by medical institutions have the budget, mandate, or skills to operate routine, sophisticated undercover surveillance; or, the technical know-how to monitor the myriad of sensitive locations within such facilities. Such is the bitter pill of our modern health care infrastructure—but an especially hard one to swallow considering the large number of dangerous drugs and the dense population of virtually helpless citizens housed within hospitals and related facilities at any given time. Furthermore, considering the irreplaceable value of medical institutions to our national health—and to our national security in a time of crisis—it is unconscionable that such a gaping hole in the defense of our nation's assets remains so open to attack.

Many elected officials and law-enforcement workers were consulted in the writing of this book. To a person, there was not one who wanted to go on the record with such frightening facts about our society's vulnerability to assault on our health care infrastructure. Sadly, one of our nation's best-kept secrets is keeping the public ignorant of "how much is just not done" when it comes to national security. All we have to do to appreciate this point is to reflect on how many years have lapsed since the Congressional bipartisan 9/11 Commission Report and the full implementation of its recommendations. The good news is that we are not completely without hope. When it comes to health care security, education and staff-driven personal surveillance (using our own "eyes and ears" at the level of the bedside) is probably the best solution to most of our security lapses. The key is to know where our most vulnerable health care "spots" lie, and to know what to look for.

ASSESSING RISKS IN THE HEALTH CARE INSTITUTION

No amount of infant security measures, basic "perimeter" access monitoring, or closed-circuit television cameras will prevent terrorism from striking American health care sites. These security steps represent the basic—and, unfortunately, the only—forms of safety afforded to most medical facilities. In our times of cost containment, this minimum level of security could be accepted if only the increased threat of terrorism were not present. The risks we *should* be gauging and preparing for in our medical institutions include the following, in progressive order of complexity and danger:

Unruly (openly disruptive) behavior is that which infringes on the safety and rights of patients, staff, and visitors. This can be handled by constant monitoring of security cameras and a minimally acceptable number of security officers. The patrol and station of the "campus police" should never exclude geographic areas that are contiguous and/or physically present on the facility grounds—i.e., parks, parking lots, walkways, and roads should all be monitored in some way.

Campus security does not need to be armed with firearms, but communication systems and protocols need to be sophisticated enough to pick up disruptions in standard operating procedure (e.g., the failure of a routine "call-in" by a peripheral unit should be treated as a serious incident until proven otherwise). The campus patrols should be able to handle both the challenge of improper human behavior and the obvious or reported theft of personnel property, facility property, and drugs/medical supplies.

Kidnapping is the purposeful or inadvertent movement of infants and minor children (or any person) from their proper location to any other place. This category is a rare exception in the realm of health care security in that kidnapping risks are fairly well controlled in hospital settings. Fears of lawsuits and public outrage have upped the standard on maternity and children's floors to include manned patrols, continuous video surveillance, alarmed doors, and matching parental and child wristbands (that trigger alarms outside of an accepted perimeter). In addition, a heightened level of vigilance on the part of nurses and other staff in this area sets an example that should be replicated in other health care settings.

Entrance/Exit Monitoring is the use of metal detectors, personnel and baggage inspection, and hidden radio-frequency identification (RFID) monitors (to detect property theft—similar to the process in department stores). This technology should be present throughout medical institutions. This would not only preclude (or decrease) the inappropriate flow of materials in and out of facilities, but also would keep better tabs on equipment and supply theft. This is certainly not done at most medical facilities across the country.

Computer/Informational Technology (IT) Monitoring is the use of electronic technology to coordinate and integrate the flow of information into, within, and out of medical facilities in an effort that is synergistic with security objectives. More and more institutions are utilizing sophisticated computer technology, 24-hour "help lines" and the latest in firewall and virus-detection software, but their use is primarily designed to detect and prevent "computer bugs" that could incapacitate a computer network. Increases in IT budgets have paralleled government-mandated requirements for insuring the privacy of patient data. Ideally, computer networks are utilized to centralize and store information related to security monitors, intrusion detection, silent "trip-wire" sensors, and employee work patterns. The electronic-age technology potentially available to medical facilities is not being fully exploited. If the preceding risk assessment variables are properly contained, other related threats—such as arson, sabotage, general vandalism, and natural disasters—will be more effectively contained.

Present-day technology allows computer-analyzed video of personnel movement within a facility to be analyzed and assessed for potential risk. This is only one example of valuable technology that is not being used on health care campuses. It is not enough for hospitals and related medical facilities to simply comply with legislative statutes as they are passed; likewise, compliance with the Joint Commission on Accreditation of Healthcare Organizations (JCAHO) standards represents only the very basic of necessary security measures (as will be detailed in Chapter 8). A proper assessment of any medical facility's potential security risks entails a basic foundation of protective measures upon which an integrated and individualized web of surveillance is built. Multiple areas need to be covered in putting together a complete picture of facility risk. The following need to be addressed/collected:

1. Detailed records of sensitive physical plant "objects," such as oxygen storage tanks, central HVAC systems, intake vents, loading docks, central water valves, fire escape portals, rooftop access, proximity to other buildings; in addition, storage locations for medications, IV fluids, and food must be identified.
2. A complete record of existing employees, new hires, behavioral reports, unusual observations, or requests by doctors, nurses, or other staff. Background investigations should be completed on all health care employees.
3. Existing security protocols and drills, as well as any security training activities performed.
4. A history of on-campus *and* neighborhood theft patterns.
5. A complete record of hours of operation and protocols for the locking and unlocking of all facility doors, entrances, and supply docks.
6. A description of procedures and practices in the process of creating and monitoring employee ID- badges; an understanding of how visitors are identified and tracked within the institution (assuming this is done at all).
7. A file of all security cameras, including an assessment of all medication, IV fluids, and other medical supply storage locations on a floor-by-floor basis. (Also, a record of what, if any, of these locations is under video surveillance and what is the procedure for the review of these tapes.)
8. A record (and organizational tracking mechanism) for every key that opens every door, cabinet, and file on the premises.

These questions are but the beginning of any security assessment, and paint a necessary "picture" of an institution in terms of risks and needs.

ESSENTIAL SECURITY MEASURES

The basic, initial change that any health care facility should implement in creating a revamped, more secure institution is the standardization of "access cards" and keys. Every individual (including visitors) in the facility should be required to use devices that allow selective entry to various locations; these devices should insure that all movements and activities could be electronically tracked. Visitors should be issued special, more restricted ID cards that likewise create an electronic "trail" and allow central security personnel to know where each person is at all times. Visitors should be required to show reliable forms of identification (drivers cards would be an acceptable form) that are then recorded in the permanent security record and tied to the temporary identification (ID) card given at the door. The ID cards should be given in exchange for an item of personal identification (e.g., driver's license) and returned when the individual permanently exits through the same site of entry. Employees with access that allow entry to drug dispensing machines, cabinets, and storage rooms should be identified by electronic clearance. The facility can program this clearance to be granted from the worker's ID badge, but should also complement this security requirement with additional technology for sensitive locations. Upgraded layers of technology can include facial recognition or fingerprint readers. All high-security locations should be under video surveillance. Even if breaches in security cannot be detected in advance, the video record allows pieces of the "puzzle" to be solved at a later time. To avoid losses that can occur to data in the event of a massive attack, security information and surveillance footage should be constantly and continuously stored to remote servers by way of the Internet.

Parking garage and vehicle "management" on medical campuses is routinely underappreciated from a security standpoint. Some facilities have security cameras that operate within parking structures and parking lots, and many facilities have video cameras that capture the exterior (and near vicinity) of buildings. It is questionable whether most facilities actually store hard copies of video footage for more than a few days, or whether there is continuous, 24-hour per day monitoring of live cameras to detect suspicious activity at the time it is occurring.

Live monitoring of surveillance cameras is certainly a major commitment and expense, but absolutely necessary in today's increasingly hostile world. In addition to video cameras, emergency phones should be available on any medical campus, on every floor of every parking garage; these phones should also be made available in selected, strategic locations across the grounds of the property as well. Often excluded from hospital security plans are simple steel-reinforced, concrete barriers alongside entrances, parking structures, and the emergency department to preclude the possibility of an explosive-laden vehicle reaching a location which could breach the structural integrity of an entire building.

When the technology becomes more affordable and practical, it may become standard operating procedure to utilize facial recognition software. Emerging advances in this area of personnel monitoring is proving to be fascinating. Utilizing sophisticated lenses, and proprietary software, facial recognition technology can detect the difference between the natural face and attempts to disguise ones appearance (e.g., heavy make-up or masks). The software analyzes what should be subtle movements of underlying muscles in the head and neck area.

External building cameras should have the ability to zoom in on suspicious activity, and even switch to "color"-mode during normal light conditions. Automatic motion-detection systems that can redirect camera angles and store snapshots of potential trouble spots are becoming commonplace. On campuses where nighttime lighting is insufficient for whatever reason, thermal imaging cameras are available. Newer security software programs can be integrated into the various technologies mentioned to actually analyze images, movements, shapes, sizes, and even activities. By screening out spurious "noise" created by the wind, airborne objects, animal movement and reflected light sources, these computer-driven programs can successfully determine whether a human being is present at a given location—and assess whether the movement, location, and time of day are all consistent with possible inappropriate behavior. By taking some of the legwork out of the video monitoring process, these programs can free up precious manpower, only alerting security personnel when safety thresholds have been breached.

Radio frequency identification armbands—much like those used to track medications and equipment—have been alluded to before in this text. This type of technology bears repeating again, because there is really no substitute for the direct tracking of individuals within a given location or facility. With computer software modules capable of analyzing these RFID tags—and when tags are paired to personal ID logs—it is possible to immediately detect if something has potentially "gone wrong." For instance, it is possible to determine if a given tag is displaying no movement at all for several minutes (e.g., taken off and discarded), or if a tag is detected in an area beyond the allotted "permission zone." It is also possible to know the nature of an individual's behavior (e.g., activity patterns such as repeatedly entering and exiting a given outside doorway) or if this behavior is concurrent with other security concerns (e.g., door alarm, nonfunctioning video camera, or blurred picture). Probably underused, RFID bands could provide a tighter control on personnel movement within health care facilities for staff members, visitors, and patients.

Almost all security experts and most security manuals fail to mention the two most important foundations to any successful "security operation"—the power supply and the data storage. Clearly, the risks to hundreds—if not thousands—of people within a health care facility should demand a higher standard than that applied to individual homes or single-office practices. It is not enough for security officers to be alerted when power is cut to security devices; it is not enough for the "alarm company" to be notified when a power cable is cut. It should be mandatory that any complex security system have at least two, independently-driven generator systems to back up the primary wall current. The final protection against losses in power should be individual, unit-based battery supplies that make it virtually impossible for thieves, terrorists, or other unwanted trespassers to "cut" the power to security monitors and sensors. Furthermore, the data generated by the security cameras and computer-based analytical software must be periodically uploaded via wireless technology to off-site servers. Without this transfer of security information, the ability to retrace and evaluate data in the aftermath of a catastrophic attack becomes impossible. The increasing availability of wireless technology should negate any argument that existing structures are too expensive to retrofit with up-to-date security hardware. Carefully concealed and protected wires, sensors, modules, and cameras can be installed effectively; and with little if any need to break down walls or conduct extensive drilling through drywall, ceilings, and floors.

REALITY CHECK

We all know that most hospitals, for example, provide moderate—if not excellent—security at certain locations within their institutions. For example, the cashier, pharmacy, psychiatric unit, maternal/fetal ward, and even administrative offices are often well secured. As we have demonstrated, many other aspects of our hospitals and health care infrastructure remain less well protected. It is obvious that we are missing the big picture when it comes to guarding against terrorist threats.

As just one salient example, the U.S. Environmental Protection Agency (EPA) publishes guidelines for protecting against terrorist and security threats. Using the Department of Homeland Security five-tiered advisory system, the EPA expounds on various measures to protect our drinking water and water utility sites. This type of information is invaluable to all public facilities, not the least of which includes health care institutions. The problem is that the information is offered in a cumbersome format: ranging from recommendations for the lowest level (*Green* = low risk of terrorist attack), then the next level (*Blue* = guarded or general risk of terrorist attack), then on to a more pressing level (*Yellow* = significant risk of terrorist attack), next to the second-highest level (*Orange* = high risk of terrorist attack), and finally to the highest level (*Red* = severe risk of terrorist attack). At each level, the reader is advised on detection, preparedness, prevention, and protection measures. No one person or facility could ever use this type of "safety chart" to effectively implement meaningful protective changes to his home or work environment. The only useful section of this security advice is contained under the section for *Red*, the most severe risk of terrorism. Based on the number of times the government alert level is changed, and on the generally poor state of preventive measures in place, the Department of Homeland Security recommendations are just not helpful. What *would be* helpful is for the national and local governments to systematically upgrade *all* public safety systems to conform to the highest level of terrorist prevention applicable to any given industry.[9]

In early December 2006, newspapers all over the country published synopses of a report put out by the Trust for America's Health, a nonpartisan advocacy group that advises on public health matters. The report came down extremely critical of our nation's general level of preparedness for various health care crises. Furthermore, and even more concerning, was the analysis that our nation's capital, Washington D.C., was near the bottom of the list in its level of readiness for bioterrorism. The report considered the numbers of hospital beds available, and also assessed regional stockpiles of vaccines and emergency medical supplies and personnel. The report was again yet another example of educated people investing huge amounts of time and resources directed mostly at how our society will *respond* to a disaster once it has occurred; the responses of Federal and state health officials in this report were primarily defensive. Sadly, they again missed the point. As a society, we should not allow ourselves the luxury to think of "responding" to terrorism or other disasters until we have thoroughly exhausted all means of preventing such tragedies from ever occurring. When it comes to health care (and hospitals in particular), we need to begin looking at the numerous weaknesses within our medical infrastructure and start to make remedial changes.[10]

THE INSIDE-JOB: A HYPOTHETICAL

Janice is a phlebotomist. Her job is to take a cart of blood-drawing equipment to virtually every location within the hospital to draw blood for the various laboratory tests ordered by physicians. She begins her day at five o'clock in the morning, and works until three in the afternoon. Her work requires access to the hospital computer system, so that she may gain information to the various tests and locations of her patients. Her daily journey includes the intensive care unit (ICU), the pediatric ward, the maternity ward, the operating room holding area, and the emergency room. She also visits every patient floor in the hospital. Her cart is full of clean supplies, and also vials of blood already drawn and labeled (and ready for delivery to the various laboratories for testing). Janice wears a white coat, has a hospital ID badge, and is granted access through every door and passageway. She works alongside doctors, nurses and aides all day long; most of the time she isn't noticed or even spoken to. She communicates with her patients as needed to perform her function, then moves on to the next bedside or room. Janice has never had her materials inspected or checked by any member of the hospital team—they are happy that she is performing her job and that their laboratory values appear on the computer screen and in the patient chart at regular intervals during the day. If the labs are done, Janice is doing her job and no one asks questions.

Janice is a high school graduate. After the completion of her secondary education, she attempted college but soon became disenchanted and dropped out. Her job as a phlebotomist required a brief course in learning how to draw blood, and pays a salary adequate to cover her apartment and monthly food costs. Although minimally challenging, Janice's work offers reasonable hours and the opportunity to pick up extra shifts occasionally. In her spare time, Janice has become consumed by an interest in the plight of people living in third world countries. Through her readings at the local library, she has become convinced that her own country is complicit in harming countless numbers of innocent people because of her own government's overzealous military aggression. Janice has begun to conspire to take matters into her own hands and mete out justice in her own little way. She has noticed that she is often in the rooms of patients alone; in addition, some of her patients are dozing or unconscious. Furthermore, she is well aware of the ample space her phlebotomy cart provides for supplies that can be well concealed and wheeled anywhere on the hospital campus. In fact, to save money, she has gotten into the habit of bringing a book and a bag lunch to work. She has started storing them on the bottom rung of her phlebotomy cart. If she decided to forgo these items, she would have the space to stow away something secret.

In her readings through crime novels, Janice has learned a lot about how people have been killed using medicines—medicines she could accumulate without too much difficulty while performing her duties. She has read all about exotic biological toxins and infectious agents in the newspaper, but has no idea how she could obtain them. She does know, however, that she could draw blood from patients known to have a particular disease, and then use this to infect other patients (either directly during the act of drawing blood, or by injecting small amounts into their IV tubing). Janice has realized that she could also deposit just about any device or agent virtually anywhere in the hospital and never be noticed. She is convinced that any activity she would take, if performed randomly, would be essentially impossible to trace. Most of the effects of her actions would take place over the course of hours or days after the event, thus removing her from the scene of the crime. With the high volume of interactions and interventions occurring to any given patient, her nefarious involvement in patient care would be almost invisible to an outsider. Janice was acutely aware of the paucity of hospital security cameras, and knowledgeable as to the absence of such cameras in private patient quarters.

In essence, Janice came to realize that she had enormous power. She could affect the lives of tens, hundreds, or maybe thousands of people. She could selectively target patients—possibly those she suspected had been in the military. Janice was planning to become a terrorist. Not only were her movements throughout the hospital essentially unmonitored, but the supplies and medicines should could possibly access were likewise not being tracked. Janice was a dangerous person in a very vulnerable place; her victims would be helpless.

Chance, Careless, or Criminal?

Medical care in the United States is the most expensive in the world. It also contains the highest percentage of "errors" amongst similar, developed nations. Surveys put the number of treatment errors, adverse reactions, medication mix-ups, and other unknown "mistakes" for American patients to occur in 34 percent of all cases.[11]

8

ACCREDITATION STANDARDS—LAX OR NOT ENFORCED?

Restlessness and discontent are the first necessities of progress
—Thomas A. Edison

. . . Look. They pay good money for the survey, and we work with them. If the
facility serves an irreplaceable function to the community—maybe an inner city
institution—then we're a little easier on certain standards. The last thing we want
to do is close a place down. It hurts them and it looks bad for us. I can remember
giving warnings and coming back to re-check places, but I can't remember ever
closing one down on the spot. It doesn't matter how unsafe things might be, it
just doesn't happen."
—State licensing official

On November 27, 2006, Newt Gingrich, former Speaker of the U.S. House of
Representatives, gave a speech in New Hampshire that addressed the grave
consequences which face the American people and the U.S. homeland if we
do not act to shore up crucial vulnerabilities in our open society. He received
some criticism from certain corners of the political spectrum for suggesting
measures that could curtail our free speech and First Amendment rights. Newt
Gingrich was, unfortunately, misunderstood by these critics, for his message
was rather a wise warning—a cry to action—to an American public weary of
war and critical of those who would dare "cry wolf" when it comes to national
security. What the former Speaker was saying is that we, as a nation, are
acutely "at risk" for another major terrorist attack on our soil—one that could
fell an entire city. He explained: ". . . if I come to you and say that there is a
couple that hates you so much that they will kill their six month old baby in
order to kill you, I am describing a level of ferocity, and a level of savagery
beyond anything we have tried to deal with."[1]

People tend to think that their government—the American government—will
protect them. This attitude arises out of a feeling of trust and confidence in the

institutions of public service that make up this great nation. And, admittedly, we do things well here in the United States. Our elected officials are generally competent, and our rigid standards of excellence parlay into a very effective oversight of the many agencies that lend their stamp of approval to the "systems" that run the infrastructure of this country. When it comes to health care (and the standards that dictate how our medical facilities operate, are evaluated, surveyed, and assessed for adherence to mandatory safety requirements), we as a society have fallen short. It is not that we do not care to define the highest level of security measures for our health care institutions and medical practices, but rather that those "in charge" of writing and enforcing our national standards have not examined the scope of our vulnerabilities. Health care officials need to better understand how our medical accreditation standards are lax when it comes to security. In this chapter, we will *not* look at the organizations that set the guidelines and rules for the administration of health care standards in the United States. The organizations which perform these functions include, primarily, the nonprofit Joint Commission on the Accreditation of Healthcare Organizations (JCAHO) and the nonprofit Accreditation Association for Ambulatory Health Care (AAAHC),[2, 3] various state agencies, and the Federal government (the Center for Medicare and Medicaid Services, formerly known as "Medicare" or the Health Care Financing Administration). These entities perform an admirable function and *are not* to blame for lacking stricter standards when it comes to security measures in U.S. health care institutions. The blame falls upon all of us as a society; hopefully, this book will stimulate improvements and the retooling (i.e., tightening) of accreditation safety measures.

Health care facilities are evaluated by categories, which are generically called "standards." Each accrediting body will group these standards (or subject areas) by its own number or code system—these labels are of no importance to our discussion. What are central to this text are the safety and security topics themselves. For our purposes, each pertinent accreditation area will be separated by a subheading. Of particular value will be our attempt to describe not only the insufficient nature and extent of the various standards, but the reality of how each standard is implemented in the clinical setting. Health care administrators and policy makers may have the best intentions in mind when they map out the requirements and rules governing how medicine should be delivered to deserve an accreditation "stamp of approval," but they often lack the perspective of how policies are actually carried out. Furthermore, input (and feedback) from physicians, nurses, and other health care personnel is usually designed to facilitate the practice of delivering care in an unimpeded fashion; this often has the effect of diluting security measures in the interest of efficiency. Guarding against untoward events, however, should not be restrained by a desire to get things done more easily. Our attempts to prevent terrorism (and any exploitation of our health care system vulnerabilities which could lead to harm) cannot be sacrificed upon the altar of convenience.

ACCREDITATION PRIMER

The main accrediting bodies and government organizations all look at the following categories when evaluating a health care facility: facilities and environment, governance and administration, medical records, quality of care, peer review and quality improvement, credentialing and privileging, and emergency preparedness. The Accreditation Association for Ambulatory Health Care has the option of affording a "passed" status for six months, one year, or three years, after which a reaccreditation survey is necessary. The approximate cost of a full three-year AAAHC survey can run upwards of three to four thousand dollars, depending on the size and scope of the freestanding ambulatory surgical facility. The cost of a JCAHO survey can run four to five thousand dollars for a free-standing surgery center, and over ten thousand dollars (or more) for a large in-patient hospital settings. Three-year accreditation terms are granted by JCAHO, unless gross deficiencies are detected and limited; temporary extensions of existing approvals are afforded pending further investigation or resurvey. The issue of accreditation status may be extremely touchy to facility administrators—and great efforts may be made to politically mitigate any deficient evaluations—because both Federal and state money and insurance reimbursement are usually contingent upon receiving a passing grade. The other main, independent entity which accredits office-based, primarily plastic surgery operating rooms is called American Association for Accreditation of Ambulatory Surgical Facilities, Inc. (AAAASF).[4] The AAAASF survey process grants three-year terms of accreditation and costs approximately one thousand dollars.

Regarding nonhospital medical/surgical entities, JCAHO and AAAHC will not grant accreditation in states where licensure of the facility is also required unless the organization has gone through the licensure process as well. The AAAASF does not require state licensure. This difference may seem trivial, until it is appreciated that AAAASF-accredited facilities may not have physical plant and emergency-response measures in place to meet even the most basic of state-required standards.

PATIENT-ORIENTED: THE STANDARD OF ACCURACY IN PATIENT (AND PRODUCT) IDENTIFICATION

This category (or set of standards) of patient-oriented safety measures is designed to prevent the wrong procedure being performed on a patient; it also serves to prevent the wrong blood product or medication being delivered to a patient. Various guidelines and protocols have been created to "time out" before procedures and surgeries, insuring that an active communication process is in place amongst all the health care providers present (as well as the patient). By following a rigid, repetitive process before a patient undergoes a medical procedure or surgery, all health care personnel make sure that they are "on the same page" so that there is no misunderstanding or confusion about what is to transpire. This practice is excellent and should not be changed.

We begin to see the empty nature of this set of standards, however, as they are applied to the delivery of blood products and medications. The standards demand that at least two patient identifiers are used to "zero in" on the correct patient and the correct product. The patient room number cannot be used as an identifier. For example, products that are generated by the blood bank or pharmacy will come to the bedside or operating table with a label. This label will be cross-checked with the patient wrist band to confirm that the patient name, date of birth, medical record number, and attending physician of record all match. In addition, the physician order sheet (and accompanying product paperwork) is checked to insure that the product codes, descriptions, date of preparation, date of expiration, and any other identifiers are all exactly the same. Blood products come with various identification codes and numbers and these must be perfectly matched. Before administration of blood products, even in emergency situations, two health care professionals (e.g., a physician and a registered nurse) must sign off on the product to be delivered to the patient. With regard to the delivery of medications at the bedside, all that is required is that the syringe or bottle of medicine be labeled with the medicine name, the patient name, the date and time of preparation (i.e., if the product was drawn up or prepared), and the concentration or dosage of the medication. The product labeling must be checked for evidence of a valid date of expiration and the date of delivery must precede the date of expiration. If the product was opened and prepared outside of its original packaging, the nurse or physician must affix her signature or initials to the bottle, syringe, or container. At its face, these criteria appear to be more than adequate to provide for patient safety. In fact, they appear to be reasonably cautious and thorough. The problem, of course, is that the safe and secure delivery of medicines and products to patients (as dictated by these accreditation standards) is severely lacking because there are no mechanisms or protocols to confirm what this author will call a *continuity of surveillance* from the time a product reaches a medical facility to the time it is prepared and delivered to a given patient. Let us examine the steps (and gaps in the continuity of surveillance) involved in the seemingly simple delivery of an intravenous (IV) antibiotic to a patient who is staying in a room on a hospital ward.

Once a hospital pharmacy receives a written and signed request for an antibiotic (or a verbal or computer-generated order, later backed by written or password-protected electronic documentation), the pharmacy staff begins to prepare the medication. In this simple example, the medicine may be placed in a labeled syringe, which is sealed in a plastic wrapper; antibiotics may also be placed in small infusion bags (to be connected to larger IV fluid bags for delivery by what is termed "piggy-back"), which are also often enclosed for transport in a plastic bag. The syringe or infusion bag will be specifically identified with the name of the medication, the dose (e.g., 500 milligrams), the concentration of the drug (e.g., 500 milligrams in 250 milliliters of normal saline solution or 2 milligrams per milliliter), the date and time of preparation, the date and time of expiration, the name/date of birth/medical record number (and/or other patient identifiers), and the prescribing physician. Sometimes, the handwritten initials of the person preparing the drug will be ascribed to the label as well. This "filled" order will then be transported (usually by hand) to the patient location and handed off to the nurse or physician (sometimes several handoffs may occur) who will then prepare the medicine for delivery. In our example of a patient on a hospital ward, the medicine will reach the patient's personal nurse for that shift. It is this nurse who will bring the medicine to the patient's bedside and either inject the syringe's contents into the patient's IV line or connect ("hang") the piggy-back infusion bag to the IV line for delivery over the course of a protocol-driven, set number of minutes.

As we can see in this singular example, the number of hands that actually touch this pharmacy-prepared medication can be formidable. Although previous chapters have touched on the concern over counterfeit or tainted factory-prepared medicines, let's consider the original medication source here to be valid and pure. Unlike the situation where a nurse or doctor opens a sealed (glass or hard-plastic) vial of medicine—one which can be checked for content name, concentration, and date of expiration—our example here involves a nurse or doctor administering a medication which cannot be personally validated for its continuity of surveillance. This is extremely concerning and entirely avoidable. One must remember that most patients are receiving multiple medications at the same (or, at least, overlapping) time(s). So, if a patient were to have an adverse reaction at any given time—a reaction that is presumed to be caused by a medication—it can be confounding (and dangerously confusing) to the health care providers who are desperately trying to identify the origin of the problem and reverse/treat its effects. In our example, the discerning reader (or health care professional) may notice that there is a difference in safety levels between the medicine delivered in a labeled, hard-plastic syringe (which is then packaged in a sealed plastic bag) and the soft-plastic infusion bag. The difference is that, unless we doubt the integrity or professionalism of the pharmacist preparing the medication, the syringe is a far safer mode of preparation for the medicine, because violating its contents would require breaking the plastic wrapper and either substituting a nonlabeled syringe or uncapping the syringe—both of which would be easily recognized by the receiving provider. The infusion bag (as has been described earlier in this book), has two ports at its base—one which is uncapped for connection to the patient IV line, and another which is easily penetrated by a syringe for delivery of the medication to the fluid contents inside. It is this delivery port—made up of a soft rubbery substance—that makes the infusion bag an easy target for tampering; one which is virtually impossible to detect because literally hundreds of needle penetrations can be made to the port without recognition.

There are three easily adapted changes to the accreditation standards for hospitals, surgery centers, and other medical facilities which could shore up the laxity in safety due to poor continuity of surveillance for medications. One is making it mandatory that the manufacturers of IV fluid bags include a "sealer cap," which can be placed over the infusion bag injection port after the pharmacist has filled the bag with its desired contents. This same cap could be kept in ample supply for anesthesia providers, nurses, intensive care unit personnel, and others to place over an injection port after it *should no longer be needed.* As certain IV fluid bags may be the recipients of medication injection at different times during a patient's care, the caps should be made available and made mandatory! (Note: this "cap" concept is in no way beyond any currently available technology, and yet there is no manufacturer in the world that currently makes or markets this type of device.)

The second change in the way we handle pharmacy-filled medication orders should be the requirement that every handoff of medications requires the individual "handing-off" the drug container to fully sign (not simply initial), date, and time the container in front of the person who is to receive the medicine. This would provide a more complete record of the "chain of custody" of the drug on its way to the patient bedside. Lastly, it should be required that the person delivering the medicine attest (in writing) that they are aware of no break in the integrity of the medicine's passage from site of preparation to delivery in the patient. If there is any question as to the proper adherence to protocol (or lack of documentation), the medicine should not be given. Furthermore, the medicine container should contain a removable label copy that can be affixed to the permanent medical record or scanned into the computer record.

Before we leave this accreditation category, we should examine a practice whose time has come and passed and should be forever discarded from the way we practice medicine in this country. Namely, we should stop the practice of using "reusable" multidose medication vials. Multidose vials are vials of medicines that contain preservatives and can be used (under aseptic techniques that preserve the sterility of the contents) on more than one occasion and for more than one patient. The standards require that multiple-dose vials be used only under aseptic techniques, only in accordance with the drug manufacturer's requirements, and always labeled with the initials, date, and time of the first person to "crack open" the vial. Once opened, these medicines are stored in nursing and physician carts (e.g., anesthesia supply drawers in the operating room) until the required date of disposal or expiration, which comes first. Usually, these drugs will be thrown away after fourteen days from vial opening regardless of whether the expiration date has approached. The problem with multidose vials is that once opened, they pose the same danger as the infusion bag injection ports—i.e., anyone can access them and inject anything inside of the vial and no one would know the wrong medicine was inside until it was too late!

PATIENT AND FACILITY-ORIENTED: THE STANDARD OF MEDICINAL SECURITY (WHAT IS LOCKED UP/WHEN IT IS LOCKED UP)

This standard appropriately lays out guidelines that require all medicines and most patient products to remain under lock and key on patient floors, intensive care units, emergency rooms, and operating rooms. The distribution and management of the key system can vary by institution so long as the facility has a reasonable policy and operates in accordance with that policy. The standard becomes more rigid when it comes to controlled substances (e.g., narcotics). The problem that exists with regard to this standard lies with its implementation by nurses and doctors. In everyday practice, many locked drug cabinets, drawers, and carts are left open during the course of doing business. In fact—and rightly so—some disciplines (e.g., anesthesiology) have formally petitioned the accrediting bodies to argue that the rigid application of this standard could harm patients by making potentially life-saving medicines more difficult to access quickly in times of emergency. As the argument goes, if an anesthesia cart is locked in an operating room and the anesthesiologist cannot access his medications and supplies when an acutely sick patient "rolls in" on a gurney (possibly the cart key is missing or misplaced), the outcome of that case could be adversely affected.

Patients must come first and we must not make practicing medicine so complicated that patient care suffers; but the overall safety and security of our health system's medicinal supplies must not be compromised. For years, health care experts have been calling for better mechanisms to reign in what they identify as possibly 100,000 patient deaths, or more, in the United States alone due to provider error. What if even 1 percent of these deaths were not due to provider error but due to an inadvertent—or purposeful—tainting of drugs and IV fluids? What if an untold percentage of morbidities and mortalities have been attributed to a clinical disorder (i.e., cardiac or respiratory failure) when in fact the cause was an unknown substance in the drug supply? Obviously, we may never know—but we can adhere to the standard of protecting the integrity of our medicines and supplies while also minimally affecting the workflow of our health care providers.

Anyone familiar with the process of preparing for a health care facility "site inspection" knows that, despite the recent implementation of unannounced visits, there is a coordinated effort by staff to circumvent the intentions of the inspectors. As soon as an inspector arrives at a facility (and, of course, when inspections are scheduled in advance), facility managers begin making phone calls to alert the rest of the institution. A well-prepared facility may legitimately comply with 90 percent of the required standards to pass inspection, but will temporarily compensate for its deficiency in the other 10 percent of its operations by acting in compliance during the time the inspectors are present. During inspection times, the floors and operating room halls are immaculate and free of clutter; once an inspection is complete, halls again become congested with wheelchairs, stretchers, IV poles, etc. because it is deemed too difficult to keep all unused supplies in storage rooms when not in immediate use. Likewise, supply rooms and cabinets (and the medicine carts in the emergency room, intensive care units, and the operating rooms) are all diligently kept locked during times of an inspection, but this practice is summarily discontinued across the nation as soon as inspectors have officially left the premises and/or completed their exit interviews. Things return to normal, drugs are left exposed, and carts are left open; IV fluids—which are rarely kept under lock and key under any condition—are, again, left readily accessible in locations that are open to anyone in scrubs who knows where to look.

This duplicity and deception (a well-known industry secret) is entirely avoidable when it comes to the standard of locking medicines and medicinal supplies. The answer lies in readily available technologies that allow facilities to abandon cumbersome and easily lost locks and keys. The answer is to use carts, cabinets, and rooms that are activated by fingerprint scanners. As new employees are indoctrinated into the institution, their fingerprint is scanned into the security system's computer database. Of course, more expensive, new technologies are emerging in the area of biometrics (e.g., facial recognition software) and can also be used. In the same vein, video surveillance should be a minimal requirement of all sensitive access points, such as drug-dispensing machines, medicine cabinets, intensive care unit or emergency room supply rooms, and operating room doors. It should be possibly to review a security tape to find out who was in a given area at any time. The use of these new technologies can allow very rapid access to needed supplies in times of emergency, and will fully comply with the important standards of care in this area of health care delivery.

FACILITY-ORIENTED: THE STANDARD OF FIRE SAFETY[5]

One can imagine that the issue of fire safety and facility-oriented emergency protection will be paramount in the event of any type of untoward event—be it accidental or terrorist-related. Fire safety rules are complex and will depend on the type of structure addressed. The typical freestanding medical practice, if located within a commercial office building or complex will be built with the concept of "orderly evacuation" in the event of a fire or other emergency. In contrast, hospitals cannot practically evacuate every inpatient *in most cases*. Hence, hospitals and large medical institutions are constructed with the idea of "protect in place." In other words, fire walls, sprinkler systems, alarms, and lateral routes of evacuation are all planned in the event a disaster should occur. If an elevator is present, the elevator must be able to accommodate several assistants and resuscitation supplies in addition to a patient on a stretcher. All medical organizations are required to practice (at least quarterly) various fire alarm and medical "code" emergency drills.

One of the greatest challenges in the setting of a disaster involving fire is the issue of air handling and proper ventilation. In addition to flames and extremely hot temperatures, there may be toxic fumes. Hospitals usually have some areas of well-segmented/separated rooms (e.g., operating rooms) where individual ventilation and exhaust systems exist. Other facilities (and many areas within hospitals) suffer from single ventilation systems that serve vast areas of square footage.

For practical purposes, it is hard to conceive of burdening the overly taxed health care system any further by imposing onerous requirements for additional air handlers, fire-protected "safe rooms," or disaster bunkers. The more reasonable approach involves better use of existing resources, disaster planning, and security and surveillance measures to prevent catastrophes from occurring in the first place.

FACILITY-ORIENTED: THE STANDARD OF OCCUPATIONAL SAFETY[6]

All medical facilities must comply with Occupational Safety and Health Administration (OSHA) standards. When more stringent state-level rules exist (usually overseen by state-based OSHA branches), the tighter standards apply. Occupational Safety and Health Administration standards spell out requirements to insure patient and staff protection from toxic exposures. The rules dictate how policies and procedures must exist to address hazardous chemical risks, and how facilities must act to minimize exposure to biohazardous waste. It is responsible for making sure that medical practitioners use "universal precautions" in requiring the use of gloves and other protective garments when treating patients. The goal of universal precautions is to treat every patient as if he could be infected with a harmful and contagious disease, and to prevent the spread of disease from one patient to other patients or health care workers.

Of all the standards required for health care facility accreditation, probably none are as well defined (and backed by the weight of governmental agency support) as those addressing occupational safety. If a problem exists in a health care institution or private practice relating to the occupational health and safety program, it is because of a foolish disregard on the part of the health care practitioners themselves. The laws and agency rules are unequivocal and extremely well defined. In fact, OSHA rules are so crucial to the everyday practice of safe medicine that medical providers, irrespective of the abstract risk of outside meddling, ignore them at their own risk. Providers of health services in the United States also should know that state and Federal OSHA departments are empowered with the ability to impose a ten thousand dollar fine per violation. For instance, if a complaint is filed with an OSHA office about the inappropriate disposal of needles in an operating room, then an OSHA officer will likely plan an inspection of that facility. The OSHA visit may not be announced, and it is possible that it may be conducted secretly— i.e., with a government representative posing as a patient. If that site visit reveals an overstuffed needle sharp container, a technician drawing blood without gloves, and the unsafe disposal of a dangerous chemical—in all, three violations—the inspected institution could receive a notice of reprimand and a fine of thirty thousand dollars. Furthermore, it is possible that the health department may temporarily close the facility down and suspend its license to practice medicine until which time further inspections are conducted and deficiencies are corrected.

The general theme regarding OSHA regulations should be becoming clear— specifically, that the only improvements necessary nationwide to insure maximal protection against unknown or untoward outside forces is a site by site dedication to comply with strict regulations already in place. Facility OSHA programs should require that chemical, radiological, medicinal waste, and toxic physical hazards be identified, appropriately labeled, and controlled. Detailed policy manuals should determine institutional-based protocols for dealing with these hazards. In-house policies and procedures should lay out analyses of "job hazards," explain how these risks will be mitigated, and describe how periodic, mandatory training programs will work to minimize these risks. To insure that employees and patients are best protected, each institution should arrange for their own people to conduct announced and unannounced inspections of all areas of operation. These inspections may look at how cleaning compounds are stored on patient wards or how blood from suction canisters is disposed of in the operating room; likewise, they will check the process by which medical waste is incinerated or leftover radioactive material is transported away from a facility after use in treating a cancer patient.

INSTITUTION-ORIENTED: CONTINUITY OF BUSINESS PLAN

It should be obvious to the reader that the practice of medicine on a scale as sophisticated as that which occurs in tens of thousands of medical facilities across this nation every day requires the convergence of virtually every aspect of modern technology. From the bedside (medicines, advanced instruments) to the supply room (hundreds of different items used to treat patients) to the administrative offices (computers, complex software programs analyzing data, and processing information), American medicine brings together just about every aspect of our society. In the same vain, medical institutions occupy such a central place at the core of our communities that any disaster (inside or outside of the medical establishment; of domestic or foreign origin) will trigger an even greater reliance on the services provided by our health care system. It is thus hard to understand how people could criticize efforts, such as this book, to bring to light deficiencies in our health care delivery infrastructure. It has been estimated that roughly 50,000 office-based operating rooms exist (attached to surgeon private practice suites) in the United States today. There are thousands of freestanding, multispecialty, multioperating room ambulatory surgery centers, and thousands more hospitals of various sizes and scopes in America. These locations are much more than locations to generate wealth—they are anything but conventional business operations. Medical facilities deliver such a crucial service to society at large that we must insure their safe operations *and* their ability to continue to operate in the face of internal or external disasters.

So, in a sense, the accreditation standard (or compilations of standards) that define the need to provide for a "continuity of medical care" is likely the most important standard of all. In the event of a fire, a breach of security, or other act of mischief that derails normal operations, a health care institution must be able to safely protect those patients and staff already under its roof and also attempt to keep its doors open for casualties, which may lay in waiting outside. A continuity of business plan insures that essential and critical functions continue in the face of mayhem. It takes into account the risks of floods and water damage, electrical storms, contamination or poisoning, epidemics, physical plant damage, and fire. This type of organized disaster plan is implemented and regularly refined/tested in the hope that some level of community service will continue, even in the face of acts of theft, arson, sabotage, and/or terrorism.

WHEN WRITING DOWN AN ACCREDITATION STANDARD IS NOT ENOUGH

In January 2001, significant upgrades and revisions to the JCAHO standards (as they apply to emergency preparedness) were published.[7] These revisions were designed to improve the way medicine is practiced in health care facilities across the nation. A summary of those accreditation changes is as follows:

1. Coordination and effect of "off-site" locations for the decontamination, isolation, and treatment of contagious patients.
2. Live practice drills to simulate different types of disaster scenarios.
3. Institution of Healthcare Organization Command and Control (HEICS) to define and improve the hierarchy of leadership and control in the event of an emergency.
4. Improved data collection and exchange of information between health system and provider (aptly termed "bi-directional" surveillance, data sharing, and communication).
5. Utilization of a "hazards vulnerability analysis" (HVA) to delineate emergencies of a man-made, natural, incendiary/explosive, chemical, biological, or nuclear source.
6. Change in approach to disasters to favor "management" techniques (i.e., emergency mitigation, preparedness, planning, response, and recovery).

Disaster plans must take into account all the areas of medical care that fall under the auspices of accrediting bodies. Security and safety, as well as waste and hazardous material plans will all be considered when coordinating a disaster plan for a given health care institution. It should be clear that every department and committee would participate in the creation of the disaster management plan. Meetings established to determine the best, facility-specific disaster plan will include doctors, nurses, technicians, sterile supply workers, administrators, security guards/police, fire marshals, environmental/physical plant workers, and janitors. There may even be representatives from the community who could offer sound advice, and add a needed perspective on how the medical facility impacts the neighborhood. Questions that should be asked in creating the master emergency management/disaster plan are as follows: How will communication take place on an internal and external basis? How will patients and nonessential staff be transported to safety? What are the best routes for evacuation? Where are the fire extinguishers and what are the recommended routes toward established fire exits? How will we address tornados, floods, hurricanes, earthquakes, and acts of war? How will we react to explosions, loss of power, fire, loss or a decrement in the oxygen supply, hostage-taking, and/or major equipment failure? Who will function in what capacity in the circumstance of a disaster, and what will be the chain of command? Who will call a given disaster plan into effect, and who will be responsible for the implementation of documentation that appropriate emergency drills have been completed? These are just some of the crucial questions that must be asked in the all-important task of insuring proper preparation for the contingency of disaster.

Chance, Careless, or Criminal?

Computerized (instead of handwritten) prescriptions are well within the technological means of every health system in the United States; these have been shown to reduce misuse and errors by 81 percent. Computerized scripts help pharmacists interpret a physician's order. When pharmacists are included in the medical care delivery team on an active basis, the number of adverse, preventable drug reactions decreases by 78 percent. Despite these impressive statistics, most facilities do not use computerized prescriptions or pharmacists in an active, clinical role.[8] In fact, many locations are considering replacing pharmacists with automated drug-dispensing devices that give out medicines in the same way an ATM machine doles out money! The drug-ATMs utilize impressive, electronic scanning and tracking techniques, but is this technology being used in the wrong way (i.e., to increase efficiency at the expense of safety and security)? If criminals or terrorists were to get to the supply-side of the drug-ATM business by stocking the machines with tainted medicines, could they more easily cause harm than would otherwise be possible? (See Appendix B.)

9

Doctors' Offices Are Vulnerable

We can rest contentedly in our sins and in our stupidities, and anyone who has watched gluttons shoveling down the most exquisite foods as if they did not know what they were eating will admit that we can ignore even pleasure. But pain insists upon being attended to. God whispers to us in our pleasures, speaks in our consciences, but shouts in our pains. It is his megaphone to rouse a deaf world.
—C.S. Lewis

...He took a scalpel out of the procedure room and starting threatening the staff...it all happened so quickly."
—Dermatology nurse

If ever a megaphone were blaring on the need to be more attentive to gaps in security measures as they apply to health care and medical facilities, it is now. If we are not in "pain" nationally with regard to our acute vulnerability to future attacks against our people and our way of life, then we are in denial. This chapter on doctors' offices may, generally, address small facilities or offices; but will also apply to medium-sized suites—with adjunct laboratories, small in-house pharmacies, procedure rooms, and operating rooms. In essence, when we think of the traditional "office" where we see our doctor, it comprises a range of entities, all falling outside of the conventional hospital or surgery center complex.

If medical institutions are more acutely vulnerable to terror attacks in more recent years, then the smaller medical office setting is likely equally at risk for infiltration, theft, criminal acts, and disaster. Although smaller facilities are traditionally exposed to a more restricted range and volume of patients, visitors, and staff (and may, hence, be deemed safer), these offices also lack dedicated security personnel and protocols.

Know Your Business

Every doctor practicing out of an office setting should refamiliarize herself with the physical layout of the suite. Careful attention should be made to the location and number of entrances, and to the greater building's emergency exits. A physician should also be a good caretaker of her investments, taking inventory at regular intervals of her employees, any unusual visitors, and the use of the computer system. Routine audits should be performed not only on financial statements, but also on the number and type of medical drugs and supplies in the office at any one time.

A doctor's medical license allows him to legally order controlled and dangerous substances not readily obtained by the general public. To the extent that a doctor's medical office is less stringently safeguarded from theft, the office setting offers a uniquely "private" way for doctors, employees, or intruders to divert harmful substances toward nefarious purposes. With less oversight in the office environment, the need to know ones employees and ones supplies becomes an even greater imperative.

The office medical practice is not only a (potentially) more likely source for contraband, but it can also be more vulnerable to infiltration and attack. Clearly, terrorists and other criminal elements tend to prefer larger targets (i.e., to get a "bigger bang for the buck"), but a string of smaller targets can be equally effective in making a political statement. Medical businesses must have contingency plans on hand to deal with intruders and theft. These should be reviewed at least yearly with staff members.

Cell phones have inadvertently become both a boon and a bane to the industry of "security". On the one hand, the fact that nearly every person everywhere has on their person a mobile phone increases the ability to dial for help in the event of an emergency. The smart professional will have readily available speed dial numbers for the building engineer, the local security office, the police, and "911" (for acute police, fire, and medical emergencies). The cell phone (with camera and PDA capability), however, can also be used to store protected information of disks, computer hard drives, and other electronic devices. The portable phone equipped with Internet access can also transmit sensitive images of patients and supplies to remote servers.

If the remote risk of physical attack is not enough to stimulate a health care professional to upgrade his security measures, then the simple fear of ending up on the wrong end of a privacy lawsuit should be enough. With newer Federal laws mandating extra measures to protect private patient health data and demographic information, the need to preserve the sanctity of the physician's office is heightened. All patient paper charts should be kept under lock and key. Office computer systems should be fortified with the latest in antivirus software. Computer operating systems, firewalls, and spyware should be updated daily for necessary security patches.

The delivery of medical care in a private practice setting demands the utmost in advanced security procedures in today's world. A thorough security assessment will include the following components:

- An examination of paper and computer methods for discarding data
- A review of access points, locks, and combinations

- A list of every employee with access to the office and internal sites
- An assessment of housekeeping and sanitation practices
- Consideration of hiring dedicated, independent security personnel
- Documentation of safety risks and known inherent security weaknesses

KNOW THE RISKS

We all tend to think of terrorism as acts of violence that take the lives of innocent people and impart destruction to physical property. This is essentially true, but there are many stages toward the ultimate, malicious attack. Every business owner, on some level, could be held accountable for criminal acts that involved or utilized his resources. There could be legal implications to the injury or death that results from controlled substances or supplies stolen from a medical practice.

The risk of attack to a private business entity will rise or fall with its geographic location, proximity to sensitive government or public facilities, and the nature of neighboring businesses. Even if a medical office escapes injury directly, being a part of a building cooperative or larger corporation that neglects basic security measures could result in long-term damage to reputation. The following are some additional risks inherent to any terrorist attack or similar catastrophe:

- Loss of life or limb
- Loss of property, equipment, and supplies
- Loss of computer data, billing and professional contact information
- Loss of staff and recruitment ability
- Psychological injury
- Legal liabilities

SECURING THE PHYSICAL PLANT

Lighting

Probably the most elegant, useful, and inexpensive approach to improved office security lies in improved lighting to all structures, waiting rooms, storage closets, and hallways. Areas that are well lit are less likely to be involved in clandestine activity. Likewise, in the interest of cost-efficiency, the installation of motion detectors that automatically trip ceiling lights is an excellent first step. Lighting is also important because it allows clear images to be recorded by closed circuit and/or Web-based security cameras.

Video Cameras

With the advent of newer, smaller, and more inexpensive security cameras, there is little excuse for any office not being fully "wired" for video surveillance. Unlike the hospital environment, where a combination of high-tech software and a continuous security guard presence is recommended, the office need only to install systems that allow streaming video to be recorded on an off-site server or hard drive. After appropriate intervals, new data can be rewritten over the old, thus providing cost savings in the area of data storage.

Alarm Systems

Every office should be equipped with at least the most basic of alarm systems. Once an office alarm is set, any intruders who attempt to bypass the door or provide an inadequate password should trip a silent alarm. Office alarm systems should be backed up with hidden, heavy-duty batteries in the event that the wall current is disconnected.

Mail Scanning Systems

Some busier medical practices and institutions are considering the purchase of mail scanning systems. These devices are designed to weed out potentially dangerous letters or packages and insure that parcels which reach the general facility are "clean."

Furniture

Although seemingly unrelated to basic security measures, the type of furniture in a medical practice can alter the security risk of a facility or office. Large, unwieldy furniture can interfere with camera angles and provide spaces for objects or packages to be hidden. The clean, tidy, and elegant arrangement of furniture can aid in reducing the risk of foul play. When cabinets and storage bins are kept to the bare necessity, there is less space to check when closing up, and less likelihood that one may forget to close a door or apply a lock. This same principle applies to office plants and potted trees. Vegetation that overgrows its container is not only a potential infectious risk, but also an impediment to the security of the office environment. No matter how "aware" and vigilant staff members may be, a cluttered office will make the job of risk management that much harder.

Electronic Access Cards

Many medical offices have taken a page out of the security playbook of much larger organizations in applying security "cards," fingerprint readers, and password keypads to their security armamentarium. The value of utilizing electronic access cards lies in the concept of security "layering". If criminals or terrorists must pass through an additional barrier to access sensitive materials, the slowed passage decreases their chances of success. In addition, electronic access points keep intruders at access junctions where security cameras can capture their picture for later identification.

Identification Badges

It may seem all too simple, but identification (ID) badges go a long way toward instilling a sense of comfort for patients in knowing the names of health care workers. From a security standpoint, the ID badge also allows a quick-glance "check" by staff and office personnel to make sure everything is as it should be. Clearly, identification badges can be stolen and misused, but our minds are fairly good at registering an internal alarm when a person, his outfit, and the ID picture do not "match up."

Window Dressing

Most medical facilities with good vantage points want to keep window views unobstructed. For privacy reasons, however, there are good reasons to also keep windowpanes hazy (i.e., clear enough to allow light to enter, but more "opaque" than "translucent"). In this vain, consideration should be given to window dressing that also precludes shattered panes from injuring those inside should an external or internal blast occur. There are manufacturers that specialize in anti-shatter window film and laminated windowpanes to achieve this result.

GETTING TO KNOW YOUR PATIENTS AND STAFF

The process of identifying patients at the time of an appointment should mirror that used in the process of hiring employees. Drivers' licenses, bank cards (tied to legitimate accounts in the same name), and/or visas should be used to make sure that people *are who they say they are.* Suspicious behavior should be immediately addressed and not tolerated. Individuals who demonstrate the following behavior should be considered a security risk:

- Patients who request to be seen during "off hours"
- Staff members who request to work alone when the office is closed
- Anyone with unusual behavior, slurred speech, or unsteady gait
- Anyone who cannot demonstrate in English their name and their purpose
- Argumentative or combative verbal assaults
- Attempts to use the office setting to promulgate political propaganda
- The promotion of religious or nationalistic ideals or icons in a disruptive manner

PREPARING FOR DISASTER—EXPANDING THE ROLE OF DOCTOR AS A COMMUNITY ASSET

This book fills a needed gap in the literature about terrorism. As previously addressed, there is a growing list of resources about how to respond to biological, chemical, and nuclear terrorism, but virtually nothing about shoring up weaknesses within our health system to minimize the possibility of American medical facilities ending up as the next "ground zero." Hopefully, this book will one day help to prevent criminal activity within medical institutions and possibly also save lives. To this end, it is important that we examine the role of the community physician's office as not only a potential victim of attack, but also a uniquely positioned asset to make a difference should an attack occur.

Little is mentioned about the private practice doctor in the scheme of terrorism response measures. Usually, public health and disaster response scenarios map out sophisticated, mobile units or teams of caregivers who are supposed to mete out relief and treatment with military-like efficiency. In reality, should a large-scale disaster befall a given locale or geographic region, it is all too likely that these formal response plans will pale in effectiveness compared to the collective resources of community-based health care providers. Just as this book previously encouraged a rethinking of our plans to mitigate disaster in the aftermath of a nuclear blast (by coordinating the resources of tens of thousands of freestanding surgery centers and office-based operating rooms across this nation), the hundreds of thousands of doctors' offices nationwide constitute an invaluable pool of expertise, supplies, and medicines should the need arise.

The U.S. Food and Drug Administration (FDA) has promoted five strategies for effective counterterrorism: awareness, prevention, preparedness, response, and recovery.[1] This book has already covered many of these areas as they pertain to the American health care system. With regard to the office-based physician, there is a great deal that can be done at the level of the community. The following represent items that could potentially be present in doctors' offices (and raise the question of whether Federal, state, and private corporation grants should be promoted to fund these supplies)[2]:

- Medical grade syringes and needles (used to draw blood and also administer life saving medications)
- Pyridostigmine tablets (treats Soman nerve gas exposure)
- Redline alert test (detects anthrax infection)
- AtroPen autoinjector (contains atropine; treats nerve gas exposure
- ThyroSafe tablets (Potassium iodide to protect against radiation damage to thyroid)
- Skin exposure reduction paste (treats exposure to blister and nerve agents)
- Ciprofloxacin and doxycycline tablets (treat post-anthrax exposure)
- Reactive skin decontamination lotion (removes chemicals and fungal toxins)

What to Do Once an Attack or Breach of Security Has Already Been Set into Motion

In the event of an attack or breach or security of any kind, one should, of course, first attend to serious personal injuries and then survey the landscape to triage injured parties and deliver needed medical care. If necessary, use a cell phone to call "911." In the event of fire, know where the nearest fire extinguisher is located and extinguish any residual flames as deemed feasible and appropriate. If there is any question of biological, chemical, or radiological contamination, it is best to await the specialized services of emergency medical personnel. Good judgment will have to guide the appropriate handling of the disaster scene, and whether it is best to simply extricate oneself immediately from the premises. In cases where toxins or airborne infectious agents may be present, it would be best to disable air handling/ventilation systems. Remember that if power is still intact, computers should be turned off to eliminate the action of their internal fans.

If a bomb threat is called in, it is of the utmost importance for the phone call recipient to obtain and recall as much information as possible from the conversation. The person calling in the threat will likely know exactly what information he wants to impart, but the individual on the facility end should try to get as much information about the planned incident (i.e., location, timing, and device) and the alleged reason (e.g., political, religious, and name of organization) as possible. While collecting information, writing notes, and trying to quietly get the attention of others in the office, it is important to make note of the caller's accent, perceived sex, age, and any other linguistic peculiarities. Other sounds picked up during the call may prove essential to stopping an attack. One should think about static or loud background noise that may imply the caller was in a car or on a roadside. Other noises may reveal animals, individuals nearby, background music, or distinctive machinery. Every piece of information is potentially a valuable clue toward the goal of saving lives. It is important to record the caller's digital phone number, retrieve the number through the assistance of the phone operator, or utilize the immediate call-back mechanism of * 57 or your carrier's applicable call trace code. Even if the caller does not seem to be serious or credible, the police should be notified by way of "911."

FOUR STEPS TO A SAFER MEDICAL OFFICE

Doctor Dorin's Four-Point Security Formula

The successful strategy for achieving a safer medical office requires assimilating known examples of security threats to medical establishments, and putting them together in a way that is practically and economically feasible. The following "four steps" cannot be found elsewhere in this context. Hopefully, these simple recommendations will be accepted on a wide scale.

---

1. Advertise and Implement Video Surveillance

Doctors' offices should be routinely built with in-house video surveillance. This surveillance should be advertised on the entrance door, apprising patients and visitors that they will be "on camera." As has been the recent practice of some bank branches, patients should be able to view themselves on a small closed circuit television as they enter the office premises. The video setup does not have to be intimidating, and it should be made clear that patient privacy was not at risk of being compromised. Patients should be informed that video images would be destroyed on a regular basis and served to protect patients and staff against unsafe behavior or intrusion. Patients should be asked to have their pictures taken so that confidential paper and/or computer files would have the photographs attached to the medical record. In the event that drug-seeking or other criminal behavior were to be identified, the photograph record could prove valuable in the course of sorting out matters of legal significance.

2. Run Background Checks on Employees

It is now considered routine for nursing homes, day care centers, and other sensitive job centers to require a several week "vetting" protocol for new employees. This process includes an FBI fingerprint analysis. This sort of background check has become "standard operating procedure" even for state real estate licensing boards. Many state medical boards require fingerprint tests as a part of the initial licensure application—and for good reason. The rigorous and intimate nature of medical practice requires that every safety precaution be taken when it comes to hiring new employees. Aside from patient safety issues, the ready exposure to controlled and dangerous substances makes fingerprint checks a prudent measure.

3. "Score" Office Medicine Vials and Supplies

Every medical practice will have different types of drugs and supplies. Some, such as chronic pain practices, will store large quantities of painkillers; other practices may have only minimal supplies of local anesthetics and wound dressings. Regardless of the type of office practice, every practitioner will want to insure that her inventory remains intact and free of theft. One inexpensive way to protect office supplies and make sure they are not diverted for other uses, is to personally "score" or mark every box, package, vial, and item once it is received from the factory or supply representative. For example, medicine vials should be marked with bright colored or fluorescent permanent markers to let anyone who might see the product outside of the private office that it is out of place.

4. Get State Medical Boards or Societies to Form Web-Based "Alert" Systems

State medical boards already require physicians to register with valid office and personal E-mail addresses. This database allows the organizations to easily disseminate information, provide for licensure or membership renewals, and gather personnel in the event it is required for disaster response plans. Utilizing these existing networks, doctors should work to have their respective medical representatives form regional Web-based "alert" systems. Specifically, the alerts or bulletins would pass on information by members regarding criminal activity, thefts, or other suspicious patterns through periodic electronic mailings. For example, if a state medical board was notified that a suspicious individual was attempting to pass himself off as a drug supply representative to various medical offices within the same geographic area—and this data was reviewed by law enforcement officials as being credible—the board could use the network of providers to warn the entire database of health care providers. In this way, a wall of defense will have been created at the level of patient care. By bringing the onus of providing security to the health care system "in-house," rather than by relying solely on community-based law enforcement officials, the medical establishment will be raising the bar of safety when it comes to terrorism prevention.

STAFF TRAINING AND COMPETENCY

Like hospital employees, medical office workers should be held to a level of training and competency that reflects reasonable community standards. With regard to terrorism prevention—and a strengthening of the weaknesses in the way health care is delivered in this country—we need to expect the highest level of attention and commitment to safety and security concerns.

Health care professionals and medical support staff, in all clinical settings, should be tested annually on such diverse issues as billing compliance, occupational hazards, emergency medical management, and lab safety. An essential area of review is the subject of handling sensitive (personal) patient information and data. In 1996, the U.S. Department of Health and Human Services issued Health Insurance Portability and Accountability Act (HIPAA) rules.[3] These rules address the importance of patient privacy rights and the need to insure that sensitive records remain confidential.

In the area of disaster preparedness and prevention, it is important to remember how integral the medical office setting is in relation to the overall community health care system. As a result of the vast resources (and potentially harmful agents and tools), which exist at medical office practices, the individual practitioner must be mindful of his responsibility to both offer help when needed and exercise reasonable safeguards over his practice inventory. Disaster plans, mock "codes," radiation safety drills, and fire drills should be conducted *at the very minimum* annually. Mandatory in-house training should be conducted for blood-borne pathogens, hazardous chemicals, and communicable disease transmission prevention. Risk management activities would be well to include policies for integrating into local disaster response/management plans should the situation arise.

A WORD ABOUT MANAGING RISK

Anyone can put together a list of tragedies that have befallen human beings in any culture and period of history. And, we can all fall into the trap of feeling like the "big" institution (read hospital, university, and health system) will ultimately protect us when it comes to managing professional risks. The truth is that human nature and common human experience should tell us otherwise. We do not need statistics or scientific references to personally validate the reality that people will generally do the least amount necessary in any given area of life to achieve the desired goal. Perhaps this behavior is adaptive from some evolutionary paradigm to preserve energy in the rare, but potentially life-saving, setting of reacting to external threats; maybe, it is simply a part of our God-given "nature." Nevertheless, this pattern of behavior is anything but protective or adaptive in the modern world, where threats and disasters seem to be becoming all too frequent. If we can find a way to minimize risks—and hence *prevent* bad events from occurring in the first place, then possibly we can truly improve the quality of our daily lives.

In his excellent paper, "Disaster Medicine in the 21st Century: Future Hazards, Vulnerabilities, and Risk," Dr. Jeffrey Arnold discusses the concept that risk in life is variable depending on how we act. In his analysis, risk is dynamic; the possibility and extent of a disaster increases with the environmental hazards and inherent vulnerability of the situation, and decreases to the extent that we manage the event.[4] To the extent that we allow ourselves to step back and survey the landscape that is the modern world, we instantly recognize the elegance of this conclusion. For reasons that consume hours upon hours perched on the psychoanalyst's couch, the human condition is too often preoccupied with "false alarms" and perceived threats (e.g., comparisons with, or derogatory comments about, peers; anxiety about frivolous lawsuits; motivations of revenge; desires to accumulate greater wealth). Often the best of the human spirit rises to the occasion when catastrophe strikes, but it may be "too little, too late" at that point. From a practical standpoint, neither this expanse of thought, nor any self-help book for that matter, can change the fundamental frailties of our species, but this should not stop us from making constructive and positive improvements as a society. Rather, it should drive us further and harder to make a difference.

It is this author's view that human beings perform best when competition drives the free market machine. The need for health care safety nets (e.g., health insurance for the roughly forty million uninsured Americans) notwithstanding, we need to find better ways to motivate the medical field to close the gaps of vulnerability in disaster prevention. No amount of additional, onerous regulations will bring out the best that we have to offer. The answer does not lie in the framework of another regulation designed to increase paperwork and impede the delivery of care, although some new regulations are necessary. It lies in the power of the community health care provider—the doctor, nurse, and technician who work at the corner office—and in their ability to network with the hundreds of thousands of similar medical office workers across this nation. The answer lies in the concept of community disaster response "teams."

Getting to the next level of community safety in mitigating and preventing disasters will require a greater deal of participation, strategizing, and planning than currently exists across the board in local medical and nursing societies. Health care providers need to want to dedicate time toward learning and mastering cooperative schemes to shore up individual lapses in risk management. These providers need to find the personal imperative to seek further education and training, and network with each other to build regional "super" emergency response units.

If it is any consolation to health care providers, the entire corporate sector of the world economy is currently consumed with the task of managing risk. John Marke, senior manager at Deloitte-Touche, LLP (a major consultant organization to the Federal government and U.S. corporations) has looked into the legal and regulatory context of managing global risk. Referencing the Economist Intelligence Unit 2005 report "Taking Risk On Board," Mr. Marke describes how 112 board members worldwide were queried as to how they managed risk internally.[5] Twenty percent of the companies responded that they had "suffered significant damage from a failure to manage risk;"[6] of these, 43 percent noted that they had reassessed their operations in the context of vulnerabilities to terrorism.[7]

A CLINICAL EXAMPLE OF "RISK" ANALYSIS (BEWARE: "DOCTOR-SPEAK")

The following is taken from a presentation I gave at a medical seminar on Systems Risk Assessment, "Disaster" Prevention, and the Pre-Op Cardiac History(or, *How Much of a Cardiac Work-up Does My Ambulatory Surgical Patient Need?*)

I posed the following questions:

> "What can go wrong with my patient today?"
> "How likely is it that my patient will suffer a cardiac 'event' peri-operatively?"
> "What are the consequences of such an event?"

I went on: "When we think of cardiac risk in the context of outpatient surgery and anesthesia, we reasonably turn to the published data on the 'cardiac work-up for the non-cardiac patient'. We can simply recite these studies and their findings, or we can try to put it all into a framework that takes into account the *broader scenario of risk management in the health care setting.* This presentation will define 'risk' as we see it from the vantage point of the anesthesiologist; it will also lay out the core of knowledge upon which our suggestions, guidelines, procedures, and national standards are based with regard to the pre-operative cardiac work-up."

In defining risk management in ambulatory surgical patients, we should heed the words of George S. Patton, U.S. General (1885–1945): "Take calculated risks. That is quite different from being rash."

Risk management in medicine is no different than that encountered in waging a battle, or in the greater struggle to maintain national security. We can define it as follows:

Medical Risk = Potential Costs/Uncertain Benefits

In approving a patient for surgery, the anesthesiologist (rightfully, the perioperative patient advocate and final "gate master" to the operating room) must weigh the potential costs to the stress of surgery and anesthesia against the uncertain benefits of having the surgery performed. If, after reviewing all the facts and comparing them to the body of literature on the subject, we find the medical risk ratio to be greater than "1," we should give pause before deciding to go ahead. Of course, this artificial construct is purposefully abstract, but it serves a valuable goal of forcing us to frame the decision to proceed with surgery in a meaningful way before resorting to statistics. No matter how rigorous we try to apply the scientific method to the preoperative cardiac evaluation of the ambulatory surgical patient, our final assessment will likely rest more with the "art" than with the "science" of our clinical trade.

In defining the potential costs to undergoing surgery and anesthesia from a cardiac perspective, we must include—amongst other things—the following: the risk of a dangerous *arrhythmia* (abnormal heart rhythm), the likelihood of a perioperative *myocardial infarction*, the potential to precipitate cardiac failure, and the probability of blood loss or other operative stressors inducing hypotension, hypertension, or a whole range of other vital sign abnormalities. For the outpatient, our concern is doubly heightened, because our job is to get the patient safely home and comfortably recovering within hours after surgery. In defining the uncertain benefits of undergoing surgery and anesthesia, we must consider such things as baseline pain and infirmity, restrictions on the activities of daily living, and the very real implications of medical disability (vis-à-vis the need to return to work to make a living).

I continued, "... in the final pre-operative analysis, our job as anesthesiologists is to avoid having a 'disaster' befall our patient, and to minimize the chance that our patient will have to be admitted to the hospital post-operatively. There are many reasons why things can and do go wrong during surgery and under the influence of anesthesia; our job as anesthesiologists is to make sure that the number of reasons 'at play' for any given patient undergoing any given surgery remain the absolute lowest while under our care."

Measuring, Qualifying, and Quantifying Cardiac Risk

In the clinical practice of medicine, there is a range to the risks facing our patients. There is the possibility of increased organ and systemic damage as one moves from "low" to "extreme" risk, as follows:

Risk of Organ and Systemic Injury = Probability of Adverse Event × Damage

In other words, risk is the measure of the probability and physiologic consequences of adverse events (this paradigm is an adaptation of the extensive work on the subject of risk management done by Dr. William W. Lowrance, from his work as the executive director of the International Medical Benefit/Risk Foundation, headquartered in Geneva, and from the work of Y.Y. Haimes, *Risk Modeling, Assessment, and Management.*[8] Additional guidance was taken from the National Research Council, *Preparing for the Revolution: Information Technology and the Future of the Research University.*[9])

EVERYDAY PRACTICE—ESTABLISHING PRIORITIES

Health care workers put in some of the most rigorous courses of study of any sector in our society to achieve "professional" status. For nurses, depending upon the number of advanced degrees sought (up to and including Ph.D.), this can amount to upwards of five to ten years of schooling after graduating high school. For physicians, just obtaining the title of "M.D." requires four years of college and an additional four years of medical school. Residency training and other postgraduate specialization will demand anywhere from three to eight more years of work before hanging a shingle and entering private practice. On average, doctors of medicine study twelve to fourteen years after high school. This is a huge commitment of time and resources, and we have not even begun to explore the dozens of examinations, certifications, licensure requirements, and specialty board assessments necessary to legally practice the medical trade.

In this vain, we should pause to reflect upon the great emotional and physical (e.g., 80–100-hour-work weeks, sleep deprivation) stress placed upon today's health care professionals. To what extent does the medical provider need to establish a basic set of priorities to guide her through a successful and rewarding career? This subject may seem at first blush incongruous to a discussion of office security and terrorist risks in general. Nothing could be further from the truth.

Although some medical specialties may require more intense adherence to details than others, most involve the daily intervention in human lives—many necessitate the use of potentially dangerous medicines and delicate (if not intrusive) procedures. In the specialty of anesthesiology, for example, where each human interaction is literally an exercise in the use of "controlled poisons" for the purpose of rendering a patient insensate to painful stimuli, the comparison to an airline pilot is appropriate. The pilot cannot afford to miss even one step in his adherence to minutiae, and neither can the anesthesiologist. Both fields necessitate the use of complex "checklists" and vigilance. Even the slightest deviation from protocol can be deadly. It is this very concept that brings us to the lesson of establishing a way of thinking about the everyday practice of medicine in America today.

Today's medical provider suffers from excessive regulatory burdens and fears of legal implications to just about anything that happens once the office door is opened for business. For those providers who "stick it out" and don't abandon the field they worked half their adult life to enter, it is as if everyday is a day of risk. In fact, risk probably occupies the minds of medical professionals more than any other topic on a daily basis. Will that emotional unstable patient file a complaint because she was nervous and cried when her intravenous line was started? Am I liable because the child tripped running on the office waiting room carpet? Did my office manager make an error because her good intentions in commiserating with a patient's boyfriend over the phone revealed too much of what is now considered "private and protected" information? Will I be sued because the patient's wound got infected after surgery? These are just some of the hundreds of risk-related fears consuming health care professionals each and every day.

The challenge for the modern medical provider is to turn these fears—maybe obsessions, if you will—of bad outcomes or misunderstandings into a more positive paradigm within which to practice. The goal should be to replace these basically useless rituals of thought with ways of thinking that actually improve the safety of everyone involved in the delivery of medical care. This author's suggestion is for every medical practitioner to create his own "pilot's list" of important areas of daily practice, and check them off in a consistent, regimented fashion. The list should address patient safety concerns, basic clinical standards as they apply to that particular discipline of medicine, and staff/facility security issues. A well-trained health care professional will have little control over the independent actions of others, no matter how good she is. If a child is going to trip and get injured—despite the best precautions and admonitions—then a child is going to trip. If a patient is going to attempt legal proceedings over a frivolous matter, then a patient is going to sue. The recent fashionable trend in medicolegal circles is that doctors should admit mistakes and not hesitate to apologize for errors—this, of course, is wise and makes for honest doctor–patient relations. But this is a horrible advice if carried to the extreme of unnaturally forcing the health care provider into a prostrated contortion of conciliation serving only to appease patient anxiety. Patients must bring with them to the examination table a responsibility for their own emotions; physicians who expend inordinate amounts of energy trying to "carry" the patient along emotionally are wasting attention that could be focused on details that may ultimately save that very patient's life.

Patients can be their own worst enemies and the overly litigious climate of medical practice today only worsens the false sense of entitlement and empowerment that patients may bring to the doctor–patient relationship. The best medical providers are those who are the best at what they do, and do not allow their desire to keep "everyone happy at every moment" to steal precious attention away from the task at hand. When we board an airplane, we may be legitimately stressed about this or that problem happening in our lives at that moment. We may be tired and upset at the way we were treated by the flight attendant, or the way the pilot abruptly pulled the plane away from the terminal in preparation for taxing down the runway and taking off. We may even feel compelled to write a letter of complaint about our experience. The most professional and successful pilot, however, will maintain focus on his job and on those things that he can control.

A successful working "safety" checklist for the office health care provider should include the following at the start and end of everyday:

1. Alarms, sensors, cameras and/or locks intact/functioning
2. Computer firewalls, antiviral software, privacy screens in place
3. Waiting room, examination rooms, labs, restroom neat/clean
4. Sterile items properly prepared and ready
5. Sensitive patient charts/records stowed away from visitor sight or access
6. Needle/sharp containers available and properly opened (not full)
7. Emergency supply inventory checked, up-to-date, and accessible
8. Drug expiration dates not exceeded
9. Drug or specimen refrigerators functioning at correct temperature

This list could go on to include dozens of other important items pertinent to a particular medical practice. The important thing is that the provider has *a list*, and adheres to a standard way of doing business that keeps him focused on the important aspects of doing the best and safest job possible. If medical professionals kept keener focus on the things they could control— rather than the overwhelming stimuli of things they have virtually no control over—they would probably find that working is more enjoyable; they might even discover new and better ways to practice. In this way, if disaster should strike and catastrophes should unfold, the health care professional is prepared and confident that everything he could have done to prevent, mitigate and/or handle the crisis has been addressed. The rest of the scenario just involves "getting through" the event and surviving to see another day. On both the big and small scale, bad things do happen in life. How we fare when tragedy occurs—on a professional and personal level—is often as much a matter of how we've lived our lives up to that point as it is a matter of fate.

Chance, Careless, or Criminal?

The U.S. FDA, charged with tracking the safety of medical devices, receives approximately 4,000 reports per year of deaths caused by faulty machines used in the health care setting. According to the FDA, this number represents a gross underrepresentation of the actual injuries caused by medical devices in any given year.[10]

10

WHAT WE CAN DO AND MUST DO STAT (ANTIDOTES AND ANECDOTES)

The American, by nature, is optimistic. He is experimental, an inventor and a builder who builds best when called upon to build greatly.

—John F. Kennedy

... They dropped us in the desert and said "build a hospital" ... So, we did just that. We popped our tents, unloaded our supplies, and worked through the night. By the next morning, we were ready to operate. Our first patient was one of our own doctors who had impaled his leg with a rod used to plant stakes deep into the sand ... We didn't know when the real Hell would fall upon us, but we were ready ... we were ready.

—Medical corpsman (Army)

The question has never been one of whether we Americans *could* do what is necessary to prepare and prevent attacks against our health care infrastructure, but whether we *would* do what was necessary to achieve that goal. The first step in becoming better prepared is to acknowledge the vulnerabilities that exist within our medical system; the second step is putting together the pieces of a successful plan. This chapter will detail those "pieces" required for adequately securing our medical establishments, and will pull together many of the concepts heretofore identified in the previous sections of this text. Where appropriate, anecdotes will be offered to round out the discussion and apply real-life context to the challenges ahead.

In his chapter on the "Implications for Military Medicine and Mass-Casualty Anesthesia,"[1] Joel W. McMaster, M.D., MAJ, MC, USA, describes the success of utilizing innovative techniques and lightweight supplies to effectively treat injured soldiers in the battlefield. Carrying on the theme of the medical textbook *Anesthesia in Cosmetic Surgery* (editor Barry L. Friedberg, M.D., 2007), McMaster details methods of anesthetizing patients that require the bare minimum of intravenous (IV) line access, only a syringe or two, and a few vials of medication. Gone from his arsenal of supplies are the heavy, unwieldy anesthesia machine and hundreds of dollars of items previously considered necessary to render patients safely "asleep" (without pain or awareness) for surgery. This clinical example is mentioned because it represents a core principle in shoring up our deficiencies and vulnerabilities to sabotage within medical settings here at home. Namely, that there are ways to do things better, if only we are willing to think in broader terms and accept changes to how we deliver medical care.

How We Practice Is How We Were Trained

In 2003, the Saint Louis University School of Nursing began a unique certificate program designed to teach nurses how to deal with terrorism.[2] The university began by sending four faculty members (two from the School of Nursing; two from the Center for the Study of Bioterrorism in the School of Public Health) to the Hadassah Medical Organization in Israel. The goal was to launch a successful teaching program here in the United States for health care professionals and "first responder" emergency medical specialists.

At the Institute of BioSecurity of the Saint Louis University School of Public Health, professionals can learn the things we need to be teaching our medical students and nursing students in their basic training. The curriculum includes instruction about anthrax, smallpox, tularemia, and the plague; the student also learns about Ricin and other deadly agents and toxins. Chemical, radiological, and nuclear contaminations are also covered in detail. Lessons on "dirty bombs" (conventional explosives laden with potentially deadly levels of radioactive compounds) and other principles of terrorist prevention and preparedness are taught.[3]

The Mershon Center for International Security Studies at the Ohio State University looks into the "ideas, identities, and decisional processes that affect security."[4] Here, the mission is to "advance the understanding of security in a global context."[5] The Mershon Center accomplishes this by researching the interplay of politics, war, terrorism, and the use of force to achieve national agendas. Through an understanding of our enemies, and the challenges that face this nation on the international stage, this curriculum at Ohio State University seeks to better define what we can do here at home to shore up weaknesses in security and promote our national defense.

Other examples of American initiatives exist that demonstrate our ability to meld higher education with a national security agenda, but they are few and far between. There is no substitute for education as the principle building block upon which all further protections against terrorism are built.

Understanding Medical Errors—Accidental or Intentional?

There have been many "flaws" and deficiencies described in this text thus far which remain intrinsic to most health care institutions across the United States. Some of these will be repeated in this section of the book. Taken as a whole, however, they beg a bigger question: how many injuries and deaths are we missing? Or, more specifically, have we been the subject of malicious acts (acts which could be copied by terrorists) within the health sector for decades without even knowing it? Although this author is not suggesting that terrorism as we think of it today has been operating freely within our hospitals and other medical facilities, it is worth questioning whether more murders (and, hence, greater potential for exploitation by terrorists) have occurred that we have simply labeled as "errors."

Studies have shown that upward of 100,000 or more deaths per year are attributable to medical errors (otherwise known as "iatrogenic" errors).[6] This rate of mortality has been compared to a large jetliner full with passengers crashing every few days. The number of deaths from car crashes alone, or AIDS alone, in any given year is less than the number of iatrogenic deaths in the United States. There are many studies and initiatives underway to further elucidate the reasons for the roughly 100,000 avoidable deaths attributable to health system errors per year. Some conclusions and statistics have already begun to trickle in, which place the blame on medication labeling errors, medical management or judgment errors, and/or deficiencies in skill (e.g., performing a given procedure or surgery). None of these studies has particular use in assisting our search to decrease risks to terrorist activity, yet. What is needed is for some of the recommendations in this book to be implemented across the board, nationally. Only then will we be able to look back and see if there has been dramatic drop in the supposed "medical treatment-induced" deaths. If we do, indeed, see a significant drop in iatrogenic-related morbidity and mortality after fixing the safety and security gaps recommended in the book, we will all be forced to pause and reflect in horror. How terrifying it will be to consider the number of past deaths we tallied as accidental or error-related, which were possibly murder. The only upside to this painful revelation will be the knowledge that we can, moving forward, better prevent criminal and terrorist actions in our health system for future patients.

Consider the following cold facts:

- One in five medications in health care facilities is incorrect (wrong time, wrong dose, or unauthorized drug). (*Archives of Internal Medicine* (Sept 9, 2002), 162(16): pp. 1897–1903.)
- Two percent of those admitted to a hospital experience major disability or death. (*International Journal for Quality in Health Care* (Oct. 2000), 12(5): pp. 379–388.)
- One and a half million people per year in America require hospitalization and 100,000 die as a result of prescription drug-related injuries. (*Journal of the American Medical Association* 1998, 279: pp. 1571–1573.)

Invest in Government-Sponsored Technological Innovations

The United States cannot afford to sit idly by as terrorist, or others with evil intentions, plot to infiltrate and kill Americans. As we have covered previously, there are advanced, new technologies in the area of product, patient, and equipment tracking (e.g., Radio-frequency identification or RFID chips); there are also emerging security surveillance techniques and sophisticated computer software programs designed to better protect and analyze law enforcement data to insure that hospitals and other medical facilities remain safe havens within our society.

It would behoove us as a nation to encourage, promote, and facilitate investment and utilization of such technologies in the years ahead. As with many areas involving change and added expenses, one good mechanism for "moving the ball forward" in implementing these new concepts and products is investment by the government. This author suggests making security in America's health care infrastructure a top priority. By doing so, we may likely find that errors, morbidities, and mortality fall across all categories of medical care—certainly not a bad thing!

One way to involve the government that stimulates competition and private sector investment is to provide a small amount of "security seed money" to each hospital, surgery center, and other comparable medical institution in the country. Let's say this is fifty thousand dollars. The money would be tied to a commitment to spend it only for safety or security-related projects. There would also be an incentive to create more extensive (and possibly entirely new) safety programs: hospitals, for example, could apply for additional matching grants that could infuse hundreds of thousands or even millions of additional dollars into much needed security upgrades. As improvements slowly begin to take place nationwide, site evaluations and awards could be given to those facilities deserving top honors in showcasing the very best in health care security.

In the last few years, the U.S. Congress has preoccupied itself with many hours of debate and new laws designed to promote improvements in medical outcomes. Some may remember articles in the newspaper discussing the idea of *pay-for-performance*. Without getting into details that are not pertinent to this book, the general concept is that our Federal and state governments (and private insurers as well) would like to see the actual end product of medical care (termed "outcomes") improve. This is tied to what health care profession-als call "evidence-based" medicine. In evidence-based medical research and health care administration, policies and procedures are designed that effect improved results. For example, if one way of performing a hip replacement results in improved mobility and reduced infection rates postoperatively, then that method is promoted over others. Gone are the days when medical studies focused predominantly on obscure details or minutiae; the researchers and medical managers of today want to know what actually works and are pushing to implement these better ways into everyday practice. To this end, the gov-ernment is trying to reward those better patient outcomes by paying hospitals and doctors more money when their patients do better. Likewise, there is also discussion (and plans) to eventually penalize those health care providers who fail to reach acceptable standards of care.

This talk of pay-for-performance all seems like a good concept, except when we consider the notion that the government is potentially missing the point entirely. What if a large percentage of errors, mistakes, bad outcomes, and deaths are actually coming from inherent deficiencies in the way we secure our medical facilities. Terrorism or criminal activity aside, what if our bad results are due to systemic flaws in the way health care is rendered in this country? What if the way we're carrying out our daily business in delivering medical care is allowing enough leeway for error, misuse, or abuse that it is actually decreasing the effectiveness of our best efforts? We will never know the answers to these questions and others unless we shore up weaknesses within the fabric of our national health care system. Pay-for-performance may be a good thing, but how could we possibly know without first implementing the recommendations of this book.

INTRAVENOUS FLUID SAFETY

No matter what line of work you are in, or how safe you think medical care is in the United States today, you would have to agree that the IV fluid "bag" as used in thousands of clinical settings everyday is unacceptably "at risk" for abuse. It is a plain and simple fact that the IV fluid bag remains a potential receptacle for just about any colorless substance, which can be injected into its rubber "port." If someone reading this book wants a good personal investment, then creating an easy-to-use, cheap "cap" (as previously described to protect the IV bag's injection port) would be a smart choice. The fact that no company has jumped into the market of creating "safety" bags for the delivery of IV fluids in operating rooms, hospital intensive care units, patient care wards, clinics, and doctors' offices shows how little attention is paid to the subject of security and disaster prevention in today's modern health care delivery system. If the clinical sector of health care in Western countries came to the recognition that safety devices of this sort were valuable, then the capital markets would "catch on" and we would see a variety of products made available to doctors and nurses.

The goals of IV fluid bag protection are as follows: to prevent the unauthorized introduction of substances into the bags (i.e., drugs which can cause harm long after their nefarious placement because they are hidden in the bag's liquid contents); to prevent the accidental or purposeful placement of dangerous compounds in the IV fluid bag without obvious clinical warning signs (e.g., potent and potentially lethal drugs delivered to health care settings only in the form of colored "dyes" which would "speak out" their identity by changing the clear IV fluid bag to some other color); to set into practice new standards by which IV fluid bags of any kind are labeled, cared for, and monitored to insure the potential for misuse or abuse is negligible.

Once a consensus is reached that our health care professionals need to pay better attention to IV fluids in the medical setting, then a healthy dialogue can begin by which improved policies, procedures, and accreditation standards can be instituted.

FIGHTING COUNTERFEIT DRUGS AND PREVENTING TAINTED DRUGS FROM REACHING PATIENTS

As discussed in Chapter 4, there is evidence that terrorist groups are deriving revenue from counterfeit drugs. We also know that terrorists have considered using tainted medicines as a means to harm or kill Americans. Sadly, our own recent history details many examples where poisoned medicinal products have been used to kill in the name of "love" and severe psychiatric illness. For these reasons, it is imperative that more resources are directed to the source (interdiction by national and international law enforcement), at the level of the pharmaceutical houses (to prevent the practice of "secondary market" purchases that often come at a price too good to be true), and at the level of the consumer (to improve education about Internet purchases and to recognize the early signs that a drug product may be fake).

Is there more that we can do to prevent drug counterfeiting and the criminal manipulation of drug ingredients? The answer is "yes." Specifically, there is something that can be done at the level of our government officials, and there is something that can be done at the level of the delivery of care. Our elected officials can put more pressure on the major centers of international drug crime, namely China, India, and Mexico. Laws could be enacted that would require drug manufacturers to request official government coupons for every batch of legitimate drugs they plan on producing and marketing to the public. No recipient of any medicine (over-the-counter *or* prescription) would be allowed to buy medicine—whether at the level of the drug warehousing distributors, the drug store chain, or the hospital—without the coupon itself changing hands and being validated during that transaction. No coupon, no drug sale. Coupon numbers would be audited and only those "in circulation" would be valid. Counterfeiters could churn out millions of fake pills a day, but their ability to sell their products in the United States at the corporate level would be severely restricted. The next step would be to prevent any Internet businesses from selling drugs to Americans without being evaluated and approved by the U.S. Food and Drug Administration (FDA). Consumers would also be advised that purchasing medicine from illegitimate sources is illegal.

At the level of the delivery of medical care, there is also a clever way to at least decrease the potential for tainted drugs reaching patients. This would require a small expense (one which could possibly be supported by government grants), but would be entirely worth the effort. The idea is to actually survey anywhere from 1 to 5 percent (for example) of the actual medicines reaching hospitals before they are dispensed to patients. In this proposed concept, the central facility pharmacy would be required to randomly open and chemically test liquid medicines, pills, and other medicinal formulas by way of the latest analyzing techniques. If necessary, samples would be sent off to regional labs for quick analysis. This plan would require that medicines are ordered "two steps in advance" of their actual need, allowing time for sample testing and reporting back to the source site. Any batch that indicated abnormalities from the stated substance would be sent for criminal analysis, and thus would never enter the patient delivery system within that institution.

In addition to site testing for medicines, pharmacies, hospitals, and other health care delivery systems would be required to electronically "tag" and track (e.g., RFID chips) every medicinal substance toward the end of eliminating theft and criminal diversion. When health care facilities nationwide eventually become electronically integrated, abnormal tag numbers could be entered into the larger database for detection at any facility across the country. Medicines that were not inventoried and tagged at the host location—or, those that were delivered without the original packaging—would be returned to a central processing plant for analysis.

SECURITY IMPROVEMENTS

The obvious security issues in health institution surveillance have already been addressed—namely, personnel and physical plant video monitoring, better observation of all entrances and exits, and, again, RFID technology to keep track of staff, patients, equipment, and drugs. Now, let's see what has been done by our government in cooperation with some corporate and health care institutions to demonstrate what *can* and *should* be done all across our nation.

In 2004, the FDA announced a new initiative to better track and protect the nation's supply chain of drugs.[7] Knowing that the emerging RFID technology would help secure not only drugs, but also supplies and people, the FDA worked with several big pharmaceutical companies in an effort to promote a sustainable growth in this type of advanced health system security. The FDA started by creating an internal "workgroup," and then expanded by recruiting the partnership of corporate America. Joining the FDA were the companies GlaxoSmithKline, Purdue Pharma, and Pfizer. Pfizer announced that it would ramp up the use of RFID tags on bottles of Viagra intended for domestic use. Purdue Pharma partnered with Johnson & Johnson to prevent theft and misuse of certain products commonly used to treat moderate to severe pain. GlaxoSmithKline likewise agreed to apply the tracking technology on at least one product line in the next few years.

In the same year, then Secretary of Health and Human Services, Tommy G. Thompson, called RFID technology an "innovative response" to combating drug counterfeiting.[8] The acting FDA Commissioner, Dr. Lester M. Crawford, called on other retailers and manufacturers to follow the lead that had been established in this area of medical security and become "early adopters of RFID."[9] In the February 18, 2004 report entitled "Combating Counterfeit Drugs," the FDA expressed its recommendation that RFID technology would be in widespread use by the year 2007. This wish did not come to pass in the short three years, but the push for increased utilization of this technology should not let up. As with many areas of the U.S. health care system, it may fall upon innovative approaches to motivate hospitals, doctors, and administrators before this type of new security measure takes greater hold. Likely, the use of grants and rewards for better "performance" (i.e., decreased theft; demonstration of an electronic pedigree or log to show a history of untainted movement of medicines within the supply chain) will be necessary before widespread participation takes off.

Success in security improvements in America's public health and medical systems is not limited to the RFID chip. Admittedly, there remains much to be done in the area of health care security; however, early examples of cooperation between community physicians, pharmacists, emergency medical specialists, and local and Federal agencies indicate that we can make a difference in fortifying our nation's medical infrastructure. One of the most important steps our communities can take toward this end is to build on site-specific alarm monitoring and detection systems. From the janitorial staff to clinicians to security guards, America's medical facilities need to be more aware of what is "going on" within their four walls. We need to collect more data, and share this information with regional and national authorities; we need to use modern technology and computer analysis programs to better understand *and prevent* those threats yet to come.

Advances in health care security can come from many different sectors. In 2001, Roche Diagnostics and the Mayo Clinic developed and came forward with a new anthrax-detection kit that could yield results within one hour.[10] Several medical product companies have begun to perfect improved gel and foam skin protectants to treat severe burns in the emergency and disaster setting. Innovations have been introduced into the industry that specializes in purifying donated blood products of viruses, bacteria, parasites, pathogens, and other contaminants; more needs to be done in this area. The U.S. Army Edgewood Chemical Biological Center and the STERIS Medical Corporation have been working to perfect technology that uses a vaporized form of hydrogen peroxide to neutralize biological and chemical weapons.[11] In the area of vaccines and other drug regimens used to guard against and treat the effects of conventional and radioactive explosions (as well as deadly chemicals and other pathogens of war), there has been some progress in the development of skin microdelivery systems as a more *effective means* to gain entry into the body. Utilizing micromolecules, and improving upon existing topical agents applied to the surface of the skin (e.g., local anesthetics), researchers have also shown progress with topically delivered vaccines against the bacteria that cause toxic shock syndrome and anthrax. In the area of health information technology, the Federal government has partnered with private electronic and communication companies to devise cost-effective, portable devices (e.g., mobile phones, PDAs) to allow disaster response crews to collect and detect harmful agents, and transmit their data to a central location for further analysis.[12]

WE NEED A CHANGE IN ATTITUDE

The problem we face as beneficiaries of the most affluent society in the history of mankind is that we are complacent. It's not that we Americans cannot rise to the challenges facing us (certainly, history has refuted this position), but rather that we usually take a while deciding that we need to take action. In the case of terrorism and the grave dangers it poses to the fabric of our society, we simply cannot afford to rely on the notion of "preparedness" for our protection in the event of large-scale criminal acts or other catastrophic events. There will always be the "nay-sayers"—those who will shoot down any new proposal in the name of impracticality or blatant laziness. As a medical director, I see these people everyday. Oftentimes, they are physicians unwilling to acknowledge basic medical principles (clearly supported in academic circles and espoused by peer-reviewed journals) because it does not suit them at the time to do so. As a result, unnecessary roadblocks are thrown up in the way of providing good patient care; or, alternatively, unsafe acts are committed in the pursuit of expediency.

In order to make a difference and prevent disaster from striking the American medical system, we need to accept the fact that "preparedness"—while a noble and albeit necessary component of responsible civic planning—is *not* the "rung" we want to hang our hat on. The only answer is prevention. Prevention of disasters must come first; only then should our emphasis fall upon "preparedness" and "response."

In the case of those principles thus far discussed in this book, preventative techniques and improved processes for the delivery of health care are also just plain "good medicine." By creating stricter policies and procedures for the manufacture, shipping, tracking, and storage of medicines, we are also decreasing theft and misuse of controlled substances. By adhering to more stringent protocols for the security of our hospitals, security centers, and other medical facilities, we are also insuring that our patients get a safer treatment environment; likewise, staff and visitors are also afforded a more protected setting in which to work. By researching and developing better ways to treat exotic diseases and toxic agents of warfare, we are pushing the envelope of innovation in the ongoing quest to find new ways to treat common illnesses. American medicine has become so fixated on modern technology driving the practitioner to new techniques and treatment modalities, that the practitioner has forgotten how to drive technology for his own goals. This author is convinced that the next level in improved outcomes and decreased "medical errors" lies in a global reshaping of the greater health system itself.

Chance, Careless, or Criminal?

Doctors report approximately 3,400 deaths per year as "unknown foodborne agent" on hospital records.[13]

11

As a Patient, What You Can Do to Protect Yourself—19 Tips for Survival

> . . . even though we spend a good deal of energy trying to get away from it, we are programmed for survival amid catastrophe.
>
> —Germaine Greer

> . . . I never thought of myself as a survivor, but I made it . . . I was the only one. Did it help that I was prepared for anything? I don't know.
>
> —Patient and undercover officer

If it has not become clear thus far in this book, the reader should at least be beginning to examine the fine line between the abstract and (thank God) heretofore remote risk of terrorist attack on American soil, and the general risk of injury or death from a poorly monitored and secured health care system. Not only do lax and ineffective accreditation regulations and a porous security environment in medical settings make clinicians more likely to commit errors, but also these fundamental weaknesses make it easier for the rare psychopathic worker to use the health care setting as his playground. The modern political crisis involving Islamic fundamentalists who have espoused their desire to kill Americans is real, but the greater topic for this text is to understand how we can make that prospect less likely within the context of our medical institutions. It is in this vain that the following *19 tips* for survival are offered. Armed with this information, we should all be much safer as we take on the occasional and inevitable role of the patient.

Tip # 1—Understand the Added Risks Posed by the Doctor Who Operates Out of His Office

On the one hand, the local plastic surgeon or dermatologist's office-based operating room may seem like a safe and secluded environment for having liposuction surgery, breast augmentation, "tummy-tuck" surgery, or even a watching others. For all of our safety, it is important that our medical institutions are under appropriate surveillance at all times. Likewise, if you are finding that you can wander around your local hospital or emergency room at two in the morning without being stopped and questioned, something is very wrong.

Tip # 10—Make Your Nurse and Doctor Wear Gloves

For any procedure involving blood or body fluids, your nurse and doctor should be wearing gloves. This makes for good hygiene, clean procedures, and minimizes the transmission of infectious agents from one source or patient to another. Simply stated, wearing gloves for medical procedures is not only the law (and standard of medical care), but it could spare your life!

Tip # 11—Be Selective About Your Patronage

If a given medical facility does not employ parking garage security guards, off-duty police in the lobby, and/or other means of "campus" surveillance and patrol, then withhold your elective patronage in favor of institutions that do exercise appropriate levels of safety and security. Most of the time it will not matter; but the one time that it does could make all the difference in the world for your life and wellbeing!

Tip # 12—Be Picky About Your Care

If you are not completely comfortable with the person providing your care, or the way a product was prepared, then you have the right (in fact, the personal obligation) to refuse that care. If you are not satisfied with the answers to your questions, then keep asking them until you are!

Tip # 13—Do Not Accept Medicine Drawn from a Previously Opened Vial

As we have previously discussed, some medicines are packaged to allow multiple uses under antiseptic technique. This can be an economical way to provide certain drugs. However, because there is too much room for error, contamination, misuse, or abuse, it is safest to refuse any medication that is not prepared from a single, safety-sealed vial or bottle.

Tip # 14—Protect Your Identity

Do not give sensitive personal information over the phone unless absolutely necessary (e.g., emergency situation calling "911"). Any information of a private nature could be used to create a false identity for someone else to access the medical system as a health care professional or patient under your name.

Tip # 15—Do Not Trust Your Health Care Administrator to Do the Right Thing—Do It Yourself!

The sad truth is that people will usually behave the same whether in a position of authority at the corner auto shop, or running a multibillion dollar medical institution. Health care administrators for pharmaceutical companies, hospital systems, surgery centers, and doctors' offices may revert to protecting their own "turf" rather than doing the proper thing in the name of health care safety and security. If you see something that is unusual, odd, potentially dangerous, or deadly, report it to your local law enforcement authorities! If you see a strange package or suspicious behavior by a medical professional, report it to your local law enforcement authorities! It is better for an innocent medical worker to be questioned about something they did not do—or for an administrator to be called about a complaint that has already been handled—than for something disastrous to happen that could have been prevented. *Prevention is the key—complain to more than one source!*

Tip # 16—Do Not Rely Exclusively on Health System "Internal Compliance Hotlines"

One of the dirty little secrets about most corporate "hotlines," ostensibly created to allow anonymous complaints about internal compliance concerns in the area of billing irregularities, medical care, or behavioral patterns, is that they are also created to keep "bad news" from reaching the outside world. This makes perfect sense from the standpoint of the corporation, because dirty laundry can be kept "in-house" and problems can be cleaned up quickly and neatly without spilling over into unnecessary and costly legal scenarios. On the other hand, problems that occur on the inside can sometimes be swept under the rug; persistent system errors can often be overlooked—or ignored—to the detriment of future patients. The bottom line here is that a serious complaint should not be exclusively delivered to the medical facility itself—far too much is at stake! Serious complaints about the quality and safety of medical care should be reported to local law enforcement authorities and to the pertinent local, state, and/or Federal health board.

Tip # 17—Beware of Irregular Billing Practices

Most people may not know that the Centers for Medicare and Medicaid Services (CMS) and other private, third-party insurers take billing irregularities *very* seriously. In fact, they take it so seriously that they feel obliged to make sure than any service they are paying for also meets appropriate safety and quality standards. This means that applicable occupational and safety hazards are investigated. The Office of the Inspector General (OIG) of the U.S. Justice Department fundamentally cares about safety, security, and quality in the delivery of health care, and will follow up on any irregularities (even if the original complaint seemed to be primarily monetary in nature). Questions and complaints can be pursued from the following websites: http://www.cms.hhs.gov (Centers for Medicare and Medicaid Services); http://www.usdoj.gov/oig (U.S. Department of Justice). Criminal activity often takes more than one manifestation within health care system.

TIP # 18—VOTE TO EMPOWER POLITICIANS WHO WILL PROTECT YOUR COMMUNITY

Few people care about national defense or national security issues until faced with a hostile foe. Few people will take health care security and the risk of terrorist or other criminal elements infiltrating (and/or misusing) our medical system, seriously until it is too late. At that time, people will realize that the basic theme of this book is honest and accurate: that emergency response teams and "bio-preparedness" is simply not enough! The only real solution to our medical system security woes is prevention. We need to vote into office politicians who share this same spirit and vision. This is absolutely *not* an issue that is "owned" by one political party or the other. It is an issue that crosses party lines depending on regional security concerns, national security funding, and other hard-to-predict factors. Get to know your political candidates and vote accordingly!

TIP # 19—TRUST YOUR EYES AND EARS

In the end, we all need medical care, and we should feel free of anxiety and angst when we need to focus on seeking and undergoing treatment. We cannot be so obsessed with the potential for inherent flaws and defects within our health care apparatus that we impede our own progress in getting well. This having been said, the best consumer is an educated one; the most educated consumer is the one who researches her doctors and facilities and trusts her instincts. If something doesn't seem right, question it!

Chance, Careless, or Criminal?

For each excess patient over the appropriate "load" per nurse, there is an associated 7 percent increase in patient mortality. With decreased resources and overworked nurses, the chance of error or "failure to rescue" critical patients goes up significantly.[3]

Patients are more likely to receive superior medical treatment in facilities that have higher nursing staff ratios; care increases in quality in proportion to the investment in newer and safer technologies.[4]

12

THE POWER FOR CHANGE—ONE DOCTOR AT A TIME

We emphasize that we believe in change because we were born of it, we have lived by it, we prospered and grew great by it. So the status quo has never been our god, and we ask no one else to bow down before it.

—Carl T. Rowan

...If I didn't think I could make a difference, I would never have joined...I enjoy the challenges and the potential to do good things. If I do my job right, I make things safer for all of us.

—Agent, Special Forces, U.S. Army

The idea of change "one doctor at a time" is valid because it recognizes that only by our own personal initiative will anyone—nurse, doctor, or layperson—move in the direction of improving upon the status quo. For change to be effective, however, we need a team of individuals at the Federal, state, and local levels working together in effecting meaningful "upgrades" to the way we do business in delivering medical care. This brings us to the concept of *public health reform.* Only by utilizing resources designed for the coordination of health care delivery at the community level will significant and lasting measures be implemented that will make us all safer and more secure from the misuse or misapplication of our national health care network. The hope is that more Americans will recognize the vulnerabilities inherent in our medical system, and contribute to a groundswell of support for a reassessment and reengineering of our health care infrastructure.

There are many ways for physicians and other health care workers to start trying to make a difference in getting safety and security improvements into place. The first step must be the coalition of willing participants—like-minded professionals who share the same goals for improvements. Ideally, entire health systems or hospital boards would create committees charged with going beyond the mere implementation of accreditation standards. From these committees could emerge a hierarchy of specialists, who would redesign the way that health care is practiced—one department at a time. In the absence of such a formal infrastructure for change, even a few physicians, pharmacists, and other health care professionals can make a huge difference by working with local medical societies and elected officials.

Once the desire to effect change is established, and a core group of "the willing" is formed, the next step is to perform a comprehensive security and safety risk assessment. The assessment should look at the available people, resources, and mechanisms utilized for the delivery of care, and arrive at conclusions about which areas are clearly deficient and need reworking. By identifying the weakest links in the chain of health care delivery first, the group can then confidently move on to fortify the other components of the delivery process. One way to insure that analyses are realistic and appropriate (and to begin to build the regional and national medical security network that is sorely lacking in this country) is to compare notes with comparable health care entities in neighboring communities.

The implementation phase of any upgrades in security at the administrative and clinical levels involves the following:

1. Education and training of all personnel in the clinical pathway; communication with all ancillary and support staff.
2. Coordination of services and changes in procedure with local authorities; instruction by the public relations department to the local community about any differences in how care will be administered.
3. Planning and execution of regular "drills" to reinforce the new methods and procedures.
4. Follow-up testing and review to insure that all members on the clinical team are working together in a concerted and effective manner.
5. Communication to local societies, the media, and elected officials as to the changes in place and, hopefully, the evidence for improvement.

ONE PHYSICIAN CAN MAKE A DIFFERENCE

If every physician practiced in accordance with the principles espoused in this book, and took to heart the *19 tips* recommended for patients in Chapter 11, we would most likely have fewer errors, happier health care "customers," and a more secure medical arena. The core basics can be described as follows:

1. Carefully supervise and observe the help provided by others in the health care team.
2. Never use a drug product unless you have personally observed its preparation from original packaging to delivery to the patient.
3. Accept prepared medications only when absolute trust exists in the source and appropriate handling by other physicians, pharmacists, or nursing personnel.
4. Avoid "checking out" or carrying on ones person (e.g., breast pocket or white coat) any medicinal vial, sterile medical supply, or controlled substance.

Medicines and supplies should be collected and used one patient at a time. The more material a doctor carries about from one place to another—or, from one patient to another—the more likely errors, mix-ups, misuse, or theft will occur.

5. Avoid carrying any personal patient identifiers away from the patient's room, central nurses' station, or medical records department. Absolutely, do not bring private patient documents home, or back and forth between the office and other locations, unless strictly monitored and deemed necessary for good patient care. This makes common sense, well beyond any privacy laws or other legal mandates. The less information that "floats about" on any given patient, the less likely that information is to fall into the wrong hands. Beyond concerns about identity theft, individuals interested in nefariously gaining access to the health care system can potentially do so more effectively if armed with sensitive patient data.

6. Encourage colleagues and nursing staff to draw up syringes and connect intravenous (IV) fluid lines only just prior to use. Premade fluid bags and medications that sit around unused for any length of time increase the probability for infection, misuse, alteration (or "spiking"), and theft.

7. Get to know your patients and their visitors/guests. Do not take anything for granted; ask questions and report any suspicious behavior.

8. Become educated about security matters as they pertain to your practice; learn about basic preventative and preparedness issues regarding conventional, chemical, biological, and nuclear terrorism risks.

9. Join local medical societies and become involved in community public health projects.

10. Question any adverse outcomes or unusual patient reactions to treatments and/or medicines. Request an autopsy on any patient who dies of unexplained or unexpected causes. In the real-life scenarios of the many health care serial killers, if even one physician had become more inquisitive earlier in the process of unusual deaths, tens or hundreds of lives could have been saved.

Accomplishing Even More as a Medical Team

Imagine what can be accomplished when dozens of regional medical teams of like-minded physicians and other health care professionals band together across this country to change deficient practices, analyze new data, and improve outcomes? The previously covered examples of test sites using real-time computer software and data entry from emergency rooms, pharmacists, private practitioners, and military installations should be only the beginning. By pooling data from diverse community sources, we can glean a picture of processes well beyond our personal field of vision. Here are some of the potential sources for data collection:

1. Fire houses and emergency medical technicians
2. Emergency rooms
3. Local health clinics and doctors' offices
4. Medical societies
5. Nursing societies

6. Local, state, and Federal law enforcement
7. Red Cross offices
8. Government officials
9. Military bases and units
10. Gas, electricity, and water utilities
11. The Centers for Disease Control (CDC)
12. National Guard Units
13. Private medical laboratories
14. Social workers
15. Local and regional jails

Ultimately, sources such as this book will stimulate enough of an interest by the public, and amongst health care professionals, that *prevention* will begin to outstrip preparedness as the most important means of dealing with medical terrorism or other crimes committed within the national health care system. Prevention can only be accomplished with a large-scale buy-in by doctors and nurses, and it will only work if we begin to apply the techniques of data collection for clinical outcome studies on a population-based, epidemiologic scale. What we need, in effect, is a new push for *evidence-based medicine* focused on the level of society itself, rather than just a few dozen patients in this or that research study.

Every medical university should require several basic courses, spread across the preclinical and clinical years of schooling (and, frankly, also into the years of residency training) on the subjects of community-based emergency medicine and disaster prevention and response. For those already in the private practice of medicine, the following areas of study would be recommended:

1. Hazardous materials
2. Basic training in the emergency response to:
   a. Conventional weapons
   b. Chemical weapons
   c. Biological weapons
   d. Nuclear weapons/radiation exposure
3. Basic law enforcement/forensic medicine principles
4. Review of the history of wartime medicine

COLLABORATION ON THE CUTTING EDGE

Two professional disciplines stand out from the crowd as being especially suited for collaboration and improved safety in the area of pharmaceutical security in the clinical setting. These specialties are anesthesiology and pharmacy. Anesthesiologists deal with some of the most dangerous and controlled substances on a daily basis; pharmacists dispense these medications and are integrally tied to the entire chain of drug utilization, from factory to the bedside. In the aftermath of the Hurricane Katrina disaster, Tenet Healthcare Corporation sold three of its medical facilities to Ochsner Health

System.[1] In renovating the institutions, Ochsner committed itself toward the implementation of advanced, new technologies in drug dispensing, tracking, and monitoring systems. Ochsner decided to automate its operating rooms with electronic medical records, and in doing so purchased the DocuSys Anesthesia Electronic Record.[2] Two components of this electronic record-keeping system are the DocuCart and the DocuJect.[3] The DocuSys Digital Medical Solutions products tout accountability, efficiency, and safety. Their system uses a keyless entry Anesthesia cart (easy to access in urgent and emergency situations; easy to lock for safe keeping), and a barcode system that scans, records, and tracks all medicines given to the patient by the anesthesiologist in the operating room. This advanced, electronic medical system creates a digital record of a patient care and goes a long way toward eliminating many of the risks posed by poorly controlled and carelessly handled pharmaceutical supplies. Another company, Picis, is arguably the growing leader in multispecialty automated medical records.[4]

QUICK INTERNET REFERENCES FOR DISASTER MANAGEMENT

Regional Disaster Information Center database: http://www.epiet.org/institutes/Epicentre.htm

U.S. Central Intelligence Agency World Factbook: http://www.cia.gov/cia/publications/factbook

World Health Organization: http://www.who.int

U.S. Centers for Disease Control and Prevention: http://www.cdc.gov

Center for Research on the Epidemiology of Disasters: http://www.cred.be

CENTERS FOR DISEASE CONTROL: A PUBLIC SOURCE OF "EMERGENCY" MEDICINE AND PUBLIC HEALTH INFORMATION

The Centers for Disease Control (CDC), based in Atlanta, Georgia, operates PULSENET, which is a countrywide network of laboratories that analyze the DNA of foodborne bacteria (commonly called the bacterial "fingerprint"). The vast CDC database serves to store and compare samples across various locations, including local labs, the U.S. Department of Agriculture, the U.S. Food and Drug Administration, international government and public laboratories, and the official laboratories of all fifty states. The CDC operates a secured, real-time online network for public health officials, offering analysis and information about suspected terrorist activities. This is called the CDC Epidemic Information Exchange (EPI-X), and is used by the Department of Homeland Security and other national security offices. Through the CDC Public Health Information Network (PHIN), multiple surveillance activities are conducted. These include the CDC Biowatch (Environmental Protection Agency data on air and water samples), the CDC Nationwide Chemical Poisoning and Radiological Illness Monitoring System, the CDC Health Alert Network (rapid, emergency E-mail system to public health officials), and the CDC Early Aberration

Reporting System ("syndromic" surveillance looking at computer metaanalysis software of multiple community data sources).

Using existing resources, and suggestions offered in this book, physicians and other health care workers will need to find ways to contribute to the terrorism preventative measures already taking root in this country and elsewhere. One of the most exciting and important new approaches toward this goal is through the use of syndromic surveillance. Syndromic surveillance simply means the use of scientific, medical, and other health-related data streams to paint a picture of an impending or unfolding disaster, when there is still time to intervene and make a positive difference in the ultimate outcome. Physicians and laypersons may think that there is nothing they can do individually to contribute to this type of surveillance, but in fact nothing could be further from the truth. Syndromic surveillance involves the use of epidemiologic clues (e.g., unusual clusters of disease, large volumes of patients at the same time with the same illness), unusual variations of common ailments occurring in large numbers, and strange patterns of disease and death in animal and plant species in a given region. Every bit of information adds another piece to a larger puzzle—one, which may hold the key to saving thousands of lives. By following leads and knowing how to be a part of the syndromic surveillance project in their community, every citizen can make a difference in ferreting out natural epidemics, criminal activity, and large-scale terrorism.

Reluctant Predictions

No one wants to predict tragedy, and this author is no exception. If this book serves an overarching goal, it is to stimulate enough of an outcry in the public forum that meaningful change is guaranteed to reengineer and reenforce our health care delivery system. The first essential step, of course, is a somber acceptance that we must improve the way medicine is practiced in this country.

It is likely that at least one, if not all three, of these predictions will come true in the next five to ten years:

The Data Will Speak for Itself (Good News): As improved data collection systems and advanced technologies slowly become enmeshed in the way health care is practiced, we will witness previously undetected sources of human error. The direct consequence of this realization will be the rapid introduction of the very points presented in this book; the end result will be that thousands of lives will be saved annually in American medical institutions.

A Megadisaster Will Strike (Bad News): Despite the implementation of major improvements in homeland security methods, and the redoubled efforts of our military and intelligence agencies, America will be hit again. This time, the strike will likely be greater than in the year 2001. The affected regional health care systems will be overwhelmed, and our reliance on a few, selective "mobile response teams" will prove to have been a mistake. We will realize that the only way to treat a megadisaster is through an entirely reworked health care security network—one that utilizes the vast resources of interconnected freestanding surgery centers, public laboratories, and doctors' offices. Let us hope we do not have to learn this lesson the hard way.

A Powerful and Well-Known Public Figure Will be Killed (Bad News): Al Qaeda and other terrorist groups know that there is only one thing more powerful than a bomb, a chemical warfare attack, or a virulent biological toxin: fear and pandemonium. These enemies know the weaknesses that exist in our free and open society, and will not hesitate to exploit them. In health care, as this book has detailed, it is not necessary for our enemies to thwart bomb-sniffing dogs and armed guards to get at highly placed, elected officials. All that is necessary to strike at individual human targets is for them to utilize the inherent flaws of our IV fluid supply, medications, and medical equipment. All that is required is an understanding of the soft underbelly of American medical institutions. Unless the Secret Service is able to test every medical supply, and analyze every drop of fluid given to the "VIP" patient, there is no practical way to effect a quick solution to this vulnerability. If terrorists are successful in this vain, not one American will feel safe walking into a doctor's office or public clinic; no hospital or surgery center will be considered a safe ground. Again, let us hope (and pray) we do not have to learn this lesson the hard way.

REFLECTING ON THE PAST AND LOOKING FORWARD

In the final analysis, it would behoove all of organized medicine to become familiar with the multidisciplinary integration of community services in the areas of law enforcement, energy and fuel supply, water sources, food storage, communications, and transportation. In the event that a major disaster is not prevented, and the best that can be hoped for is mitigation and treatment of the wounded and dying, no amount of medical knowledge will be enough to bridge the need for reliance and interdependence amongst these crucial areas of social function.

The journey toward better security in America received a painful jolt of urgency in the aftermath of 9/11, but it was Hurricane Katrina which demonstrated vividly how vulnerable our social infrastructure can be. We often take our medical services for granted until a crisis overwhelms our capacity to provide even the most basic of health care needs. If the evil of fanaticism and hatred were to strike at the core of our health care system—itself, in essence, one of our key safety nets of national well-being and national security—then we will surely regret the lack of attention paid to *prevention*. Preparedness is a noble and necessary concept, but will hardly console the losses already sustained once an attack has occurred. A strike by our enemies at American health care would effect the terrorist equivalent of the AIDS virus, crippling our ability to self heal and get back to fighting strength quickly. As a nation and a people, we cannot afford to get health care security wrong.

Chance, Careless, or Criminal?

American hospitals and other health care entities remain at an increased (and unnecessary) risk of terrorist attack, as they represent the most vulnerable of "soft targets" of our nation's infrastructure. Whether tragedy occurs by chance, carelessness, or criminal act, our patients deserve better than the status quo in medical safety and security.[5]

Appendix A: A History of Medical-related "Terrorism," Poisons, and Murder

Date	Murder weapon	Event
10,000 B.C.	Smallpox	Oldest biological weapon, possibly existed within the first farming communities of north-eastern Africa.[1]
4500 B.C.	Poisons	Sumerians of Mesopotamia (modern day Iraq) have accounts of poisons, which they attributed to a spirit called "Gula.".[2]
3000 B.C.	Poisons	Menes, first of the Pharaohs of Ancient Egypt, had a thorough knowledge of poisons derived from not only plants, but animals, minerals, and vegetables.[3]
3000 B.C.	Cyanide	Egyptians perfected the art of distillation and knew how to extract a powerful poison from peach kernels, yielding prussic acid or cyanide. Translation from a papyrus at the Louvre states: "*Pronounce not the name of I.A.O., under the penalty of the peach.*" (I.A.O.—ancient Hebrew name for God).[4]
1550 B.C.	Poisons	One of the oldest medical documents, Ebers Papyrus, contains 800 recipes for poisons such as aconite, opium, hemlock, antimony, lead. It was discovered by a Professor Ebers who saw it advertised for sale in 1872.[5]
1400 B.C.	Hellebore	The word is derived from the Greek, "elein, to injure" and "bora, food." Pliny (ancient Roman author and philosopher) wrote about the utilization of hellebore by a man called Melampus who was a physician.[6]

Date	Murder weapon	Event
6th Century B.C.	Rye Ergot	Assyrians poisoned their enemies' water wells with Rye Ergot, a fungus called Claviceps purpurea. It causes trembling, shaking, and hallucinations similar to LSD. Victim also demonstrates poisoning bytwitching and contortion of the body.[7]
700 B.C.	Hydra	From Homer's Greek mythological stories, Hercules was poisoned by his wife who had soaked his shirt with the poisonous blood of Hydra. It caused severe sweating followed by a fiery pain.[8]
590 B.C.	Hellebore	Solon of Athens utilized Hellebore to contaminate and poison the water supply of Krissa, thus causing the surrender of its inhabitants.[9]
460–377 B.C.	Arsenic	Hippocrates treated ulcers by advocating the usage of realgar paste. This material is a naturally occurring ore of Arsenic which is found in iron and lead mining.[10]
401 B.C.	Acetyl-andromedol	Xenophon, a Greek soldier and mercenary, kept anaccount of his expedition against the Persians in what is called Anabasis, which translates into *expedition* or *the march up country*. He wrote in this journal about an incident when his troops became violently ill after ingesting some of the local honeybee. They exhibited symptoms of nausea and hallucinations.
401 B.C.	Acetyl-andromedol	The honey was a local delicatessen, containing grayano toxin produced by the bees feasting on the area's rhododendron plants.[11] Alexander the Great used the text Anabasis as a tool guide for his own invasion of Persia.
400 B.C.	Poison	Scythians (a branch of ancient Iranian peoples) dipped their arrows into bacteria infested fluids from decomposing bodies and blood mixed with manure.[12]
405–359 B.C.	Poison	In Persia, queen Parysatis, mother of the Persian king Artaxerxes II, poisoned her daughter-in-law, Statira by utilizing a poisoned knife. One side of the knife was saturated with a venom (identity unknown) and used to slice a bird during dinner. Queen Parysatis partook of the uncontaminated half, whereas Statira ate the poisoned half and subsequently died.[13]

Date	Murder weapon	Event
402 B.C.	Hemlock	The "State Poison" of Athens, Hemlock, was popular as it rendered paralysis of the extremities, followed by failing of heart and lungs leading to the death of its victims. Socrates was accused of, and found guilty for attempting to corrupt the Athenian youths. This corruption stemmed from his philosophical teachings. Socrates was sentenced to death and was instructed to drink the "State Poison."[14]
4th Century B.C.	Mustard and toxic Cacodyl (Arsenic trioxide)	The Chinese Mohist sect pumped smoke from the furnaces, which burned mustard balls and other toxic vegetable matter into tunnels being dug by the enemy army.[15]
331 B.C.	Poisons	Livy, writer during ancient Roman times, had noted a high incidence of murders via poisoning by Roman high society, usually carried out at the dinner table.[16]
246 B.C.	Poisons	The Chou ritual, a Chinese custom still in existence, utilized five poisons, of which four have been identified as: green vitriol (copper sulphate), realgar (arsenic), cinnabar (mercury), and loadstone. The poisons were mixed and burnt. The resulting fumes were seared on feathers and utilized.[17]
211 B.C.	Poison	After Hannibal lost the battle against the Romans in his quest to defend Capua, the population finally surrendered due to hunger. The Senate members, who initially had favored and endorsed the alliance of Capua with Carthage, participated in a mass suicide. In this case, the poison of choice was unknown.[18]
203 B.C.	Poison	The Numidian queen, Sophonisba, takes her own life after she learns that the Roman conquerors considered her to be part of the "loot" from the war, and thus she would be treated no differently than other prisoners.[19]
197–130 B.C.	Poisons	Nicander of Colophon (Greek physician, pharmacologist) scribed two essays, Theriaca and Alexipharmaca, which are considered to be the oldest written documents on poisons. In Theriaca, he wrote about venomous beast and plant poisons. Nicander was the first person to report on the usage of leeches. In Alexipharmaca, he not only describes general poisons, but specific animal and

Date	Murder weapon	Event
		vegetable poisons. He went on further and described and listed the cures for these poisons. These essays were written in poetry format.[20]
184 B.C.	Poison	Hannibal of Carthage was known as a great military strategist. During a battle against King Eumenes of Pergamon, Hannibal's troops filled pots with venomous snakes and flung them at their enemies. Hannibal was victorious.[21]
183 B.C.	Poison	The Romans were determined to find Hannibal and kill him. Exiled and given refuge by Prusias I of Bithynia, his host wanted no war with the Romans; he agreed to give up his guest to the Romans. On the eastern shore of the Sea of Marmora, Hannibal committed suicide by ingesting a poison stored in his ring, which he had worn for a long time.[22]
130 B.C.	Poison	The Romans defeated Aristonicus in Asia Minor. Their task was not yet done, as they were faced with insurgents from the remaining army of Aristonicus. To expedite and bring an end to the war, the Romans poisoned water wells of the insurgents. They employed a popular tactic, which was to plunge diseased human and animal corpses into these water wells. The Romans were successful, and thus took control of the area.[23]
114–63 B.C.	Poison	The king of Pontos (modern day Turkey) was called Mithridates. Due to the extensive array of poisons available during this time period, Mithridates was constantly terrified of being murdered by a rival. This fear propelled him to seek ways of counteracting the effects of the toxins, leading him to study and find the antidotes. His education and knowledge on the subject arose from performing experiments on criminals who were condemned to die. He soon began ingesting daily doses of different poisons so as to provide his body with immunity. His secret modus operandi for the antidote became known as Mithridatum. The king was so fearful for his life that he refused to share his secret for the antidotes with anyone. When Pompey, the Roman

Date	Murder weapon	Event
		general, invaded Pontos, Mithridates endeavored to commit suicide by the same poisons, which he had built an immunity against. His effort failed him and he had to order one of his soldiers to stab him. When Pompey discovered Mithridates's papers on the study of poisons and their antidotes, he took it back with him to Rome. It was studied carefully by Pliny who recounted the existence of fifty-four different ingredients.[24]
82 B.C.	Poison	The Lex Cornelia was issued during the reign of the Roman dictator, Lucius Cornelius Sulla. This law or decree was the first to ban the employment of poisons in order to murder individuals.[25]
67 B.C.	Acetyl-andromedol	Just as Xenophon witnessed the sickness, which overwhelmed his troops in 401 B.C. (due to ingestion of the toxin-laden honey in the Trebizond vicinity), Pompey bore witness to the same ill-fated event. On his way to remove Mithridates as king of Pontus, Pompey's troops were greeted by the people of Trebizond who were loyal to Mithridates. They were offered the region's delicacy, the toxic honey, and fell ill-exhibiting symptoms of hallucinations and nausea.
67 B.C.	Acetyl-andromedol	Three of Pompey's army regiments, while being ravaged by sickness from the toxic honey, were assaulted and destroyed.[26]
60 B.C.–A.D. 37	Hemlock	Seneca, the Roman rhetorician and writer, drank hemlock to commit suicide.[27]
55 B.C.	Yew Tree Extract	Julius Caesar, after invading Britain, wrote in his journal that the British king, Catuvolcus, upon learning of his country's fate, committed suicide by swallowing the sap of the yew tree. Some of the symptoms, which had their onset within an hour, included vomiting, rapid heart rate, and shallow breathing. The resulting death stemmed from respiratory failure due to paralysis.[28]
36 B.C.	Belladonna	During the Parthian Wars, Marc Anthony's troops were said to have been poisoned by belladonna. Some women used belladonna (beautiful woman) to dilate their pupils, apparently, to augment their beauty. The symptoms of belladonna poisoning were described as severe dryness of the throat and

Date	Murder weapon	Event
		the mouth, a scarlet rash and the presence of convulsions.These symptoms resemble those of a rabies infection. The distinguishing feature is the dilation of the pupils.[29]
30 B.C.	Poison	Controversy remains regarding the circumstances of Cleopatra's death. It is assumed that the queen of Egypt committed suicide by a poisonous method, although the identity of the poison is not known.[30]
27 B.C.–A.D. 14	Poisons	During the reign of Emperor Augustus, it has been written that his wife, Livia, utilized various poisons to eliminate the emperor's grandchildren. There was a suspicion that she might have possibly employed the same tactic to kill her husband by poisoning.[31]
A.D. 14–37	Poison	Drusus, son of Tiberius Nero (second emperor of Rome) was poisoned by Sejanus who was a Prefect of the Praetorian Guard.[32]
A.D. 37–41	Poisons	Gaius, also known as Caligula, was a collector of poisons. He used them to kill horses, jockeys, and gladiators for his own pleasure.[33]
A.D. 40	Poisons	Dioscorides who was a Greek physician in the employment of the Roman emperor Nero, scribed a manual called Materia Medica. His work was so thorough and extensive, it continued to be in use for fifteen centuries. In it, he classified poisons into different groups: plant, animal, and mineral. He also described arsenic as a poison.[34]
A.D. 41–54	Poisonous Mushrooms	Although Claudius, the Roman emperor, has been diagnosed as to have had cerebral palsy, he was a competent emperor and managed to obliterate Caligula's poisons. Unfortunately, he himself was poisoned with toxic mushrooms by his second wife, Agrippina, who had acquired them through the infamous poisoner of the time, a woman named Locusta.[35]
A.D. 37–68	Poison	Nero, emperor of Rome and the adopted son of emperor Claudius, had a keen interest in poisons and their antidotes. His personal physician, Andromachus, enhanced the recipe of Mithridatum (antidote used by Mithridates) and renamed it Theriac of Andromachus. Instead of the original fifty-four ingredients, it now contained sixty-four ingredients.[36] Nero pardoned

Date	Murder weapon	Event
		Locusta who had poisoned Claudius, and employed her to utilize her knowledge of poisons to kill his stepbrother, Britannicus. Nero's other victims were Silanus, the governor of Asia; his aunt, Domitia, an extremely wealthy woman, along with many others. Nero even considered poisoning the entire body of the Senate. Nero's tutor, the Roman philosopher Seneca, was compelled to commit suicide by taking hemlock. The poison did not work and he was suffocated while relaxing in a steam bath.[37] Nero's favorite poison was cherry laurel water, containing the toxin, cyanide.[38]
A.D. 69	Poison	Vitellius, the Roman emperor, not only poisoned friends, but also, almost certainly, his own mother.[39]
A.D. 81–96	Sea-Hare	Domitian, the Roman emperor, was held responsible for the death of his brother, Titus, and Agricola, who was the governor of Britain. It is believed that the emperor employed the use of sea-hares.[40] Recent research by marine biologists have yielded important information on these marine creatures. They have discovered a sequence of powerful toxins from the sea-hare (Dolabella auricularia), which was, most probably, the cause for the deaths of several rivals.[41]
A.D. 117–138	Poison	Hadrian, the Roman emperor, has been implicated in the murder of his brother-in-law, Senator Servianus who at the age of 90, showed a keen interest in succeeding Hadrian as emperor. Accused of conspiracy, he committed suicide by poison. Hadrian, who was extremely ill, wanted to die. He ordered a slave to kill him with a sword. The slave was so upset, he fled. Hadrian then requested a doctor to poison him, but the doctor himself committed suicide. Finally, Hadrian attempted to stab himself, but his guards overpowered him. He eventually died from natural causes.[42]
A.D. 165–180	Smallpox or Measles	The Antonine Plague or the Plague of Galen, might have been due to either smallpox or measles transmitted to the Roman population by the returning troops after their

Date	Murder weapon	Event
		campaigns in the near East. Two Roman emperors died (Lucius Verus and Marcus Antonius). Nine years later, the disease reinfected the residents and claimed up to two thousand deaths a day in Rome. The total number of those who died has been approximated to be around five million.[43] Interestingly, the Great Plague of Athens (430–427 B.C.) struck down one-third of the Athenian population, according to the historian Thucydides. The plague originated from Ethiopia, passed through Egypt and Libya, and then to Greece. Although, the causal agent was unknown, the University of Maryland in 1999 held its Fifth Annual Medical Conference discussing the source of the outbreak in Athens. The conclusion: t it was a case of an Epidemic Typhus Fever. This disease has a 20 percent mortality rate and kills its victims after, approximately, seven days. Gangrene of the tips of toes and fingers become visible with cardiovascular collapse resulting in death.[44]
A.D. 180–192	Poisonous Figs	Commodus, adopted heir of Hadrian, had Motilenus, the prefect of the Praetorian Guard poisoned with tainted figs. In turn, an attempt was made on Commodus's life by his favorite concubine, Marcia who tried to poison him. It was an effort wasted, but remedied when Commodus was strangled to death.[45]
A.D. 250–266	Smallpox or Measles	The plague of Cyprian (the bishop of Carthage), claimed the lives of more than five thousand people a day in the city of Rome. The outbreak was blamed on the Christians who were persecuted severly.[46]
A.D. 541–542	Enterobacteria Yersinia pestis	The plague of Justinian is the first recorded pandemic which was of a bubonic nature. It might have originally come from Ethiopia or Egypt. Research has shown the plague devastated the population, costing the lives of 5,000–10,000 people per day in Constantinople alone. It was named after the Emperor Justinian I who was in power. The plague continued to ravage the population throughout the following centuries. In A.D. 588, a second outbreak of the plague struck the region of Mediterranean into modern

142

Date	Murder weapon	Event
		day France; the total death toll came to be 25 million. Between A.D. 541 and A.D. 700 Europe suffered a 50 to 60 percent loss of lives.[47]
1030–1040	Belladonna	During the reign of Duncan I who was the king of Scotland, Macbeth, fighting the Danes, instructed his soldiers to poison the entire enemy army with a liquor mixed with a blend containing belladonna, also known as dwale (French).[48]
1347–1351	Enterobacteria Yersinia pestis	The Black Plague or Black Death was termed due to its overwhelming pandemic nature in claiming lives. Its origin was in southwestern Asia, in China, and northern India, where the disease was carried by the Mongol armies along the Silk Road to the European trading city of Caffa in the Crimea (which was under Genoese rule). The city was attacked by the Mongol (Tartar) army (already suffering from the debilitating disease), which was determined not to be overpowered. The Tartar army proceeded to hurl the contaminated corpses over the city walls, infecting the population (thus using them as a biological weapon). The sick Italian merchants fled on their ships and came to Europe (Messina). By the time the ship anchored, not only were the crew members either dead or infected, but the ships might have transported infected rats and/or fleas (culprits for the transmission of the disease). The disease soon spread from Italy to all the European cities (except Poland, parts of Belgium and the Netherlands). Russia was the next victim, followed by the countries in the Middle East, from Egypt to Yemen. Overall, the plague not only caused loss of lives, but devastated the economies of the entire world. The estimated loss of lives, worldwide, due to the Black Death, has been calculated to be 75 million people.[49]
1422	Bioterrorism	The battle of Carolstein (modern day Czech Republic) was recorded into the history books as the Lithuanian soldiers catapulted the bodies of infected dead soldiers, along with two thousand cartloads

Date	Murder weapon	Event
		of excrement over the castle walls into the ranks of their enemies. Soon, deadly fever broke out, but the Lithuanians still lost the battle.[50]
1520	Smallpox	Conquistador Hernando Cortez was responsible for exposing the Aztecs to the deadly disease. The loss of lives was an astounding 3.5 million people.[51]
1532–1595	Smallpox, Measles, Mumps	Eleven years after the first epidemic in Mexico, a second epidemic took more lives. The diseases were spread by the arrival of the Spanish ships. By 1595, the estimate of the devastation was over 18 million people who perished due to the various diseases from Europe.[52]
1452–1519	Biological Warfare	Leonardo da Vinci's formula for a powdered poison was manufactured out of arsenic and verdigris. He recommended it to be hurled at enemy ships. The powder, upon impact will cause asphyxiation of its victims.[53]
1476–1507	*La Cantarella*	The Borgia family was known as infamous poisoners. The brother and sister team of Cesare and Lucrezia Borgia murdered many of their rivals by the use of a secret poison called, *La Cantarella*, which came to be known as the "poison of the Borgias." Although no one knows its exact mixture, it most probably contained copper, arsenic, and phosphorus. Their father was Pope Alexander VI.[54]
1491–1547	Poison	It is purported that King Henry VIII might have been the object of an assassination attempt, through poisoning, by his wife, Anne Boleyn.[55]
1519–1589	Poisons	Catherine de Medici of Florence, who later became queen of France, was an ardent student of the effects poisons on humans. She tested her various recipes on not only the poor, but the sick. She was extremely proficient at mixing the poisons into different foods.[56]
1533–1603	Poison	Queen Elizabeth I of England was a target of numerous poisoning attempts on her life (an example of which was to coat her saddle pommel with opium). In yet another attempt, a physician, Dr. Lopus, was hired to poison the queen, but he was discovered and

Date	Murder weapon	Event
		hanged. He was the inspiration for Shakespeare's character in the *Merchant of Venice*.[57]
1540–1544	Poison	A group of alchemists formed a secret organization called the Council of Ten in Venice. Their mission was to carry out poisoning of whomever the State deemed to be no longer an asset. Their written documentations have the victims' names, and the prices paid for the contract to be carried out.[58]
1589	*Veninum Lupinum*	Schools for poisons had been established, and a publication written by Giovanni Porta, named "Neopoliani Magioe Naturalis," illustrated the various poisoning techniques (wine was a popular vehicle for the poison). Porta gave his own formula for a powerful poison called *Veninum Lupinum*. It was a mixture of arsenic, bitter almonds, powdered glass, caustic lime, taxus baccata, and aconite. All were mixed with honey.[59]
1635–1719	*Aqua Toffana*	The most infamous poisoner of the 17th century was an Italian woman, Giulia Toffana. Her invention, *Aqua Toffana*, was a very powerful poisonous mixture, which was sold in vials under the pretense of aiding women with their complexions (arsenic did help). The vials were filled with arsenic and sold to unhappy spouses, usually wives. By the time she was executed, she had helped in the murder of more than six hundred people, mostly husbands. In 1659, she had formed a secret society to teach housewives on how to poison their husbands.[60]
1638–1680	Arsenic	In France, Catherine Deshayes Monvoisin became known as La Voisin (neighbor, Fr.). She was an extremely successful businesswoman who had become wealthy by selling poisons to housewives. It has been estimated that she was responsible for the deaths of thousands. Her business came to an end when she was burned at the stake.[61]
1662	Poison	Poisoning had become so rampant that Louis XIV issued a law prohibiting apothecaries from selling arsenic and other poisons carelessly. The purchaser was obliged to sign a register stating the reason for their

Date	Murder weapon	Event
		purchases. Arsenic had become so popular in the array of poison that it was called, *poudre de succession* or inheritance powder.[62]
1676	Poison	Marquise de Brinvilliers and her paramour, Sainte-Croix began experimenting with various poisons with the help of a Swiss apothecary called Christopher Glasser. They tried their poisons on the sick while visiting them at different hospitals (and bringing them food and wine tainted with poison). They murdered many, including her father and two brothers. Her husband, although always suspicious, died of natural causes. She was eventually arrested and found guilty.[63]
1689	Arsenic	Marie-Louise, married to King Carlos II of Spain was poisoned, although officially cholera was blamed. After ten years, the king visited her tomb and had the casket opened. The body of his wife was well-preserved and hardly decayed. Although, he did not realize the significance of this finding then, it is now certain that the queen died of arsenic poisoning.[64]
1710	Biological Weapon	Russians used an old military tactic by hurling the cadavers of plague victims over the walls of the city of Reval during their war with Sweden.[65]
1763	Smallpox	Under the false pretenses of friendship, Captain Ecuyer of the Royal Americans offers two blankets and a handkerchief to the native Americans. Both items were laced with smallpox.[66]
1767	Smallpox	Sir Jeffrey Amherst (English general), who was one of the leaders in the French and Indian War, donated blankets laced with smallpox to the Indians who were loyal to the French. The epidemic killed many of the tribes and the British were successful in their attack on Ft. Carillon.[67]
1797	Swamp Fever	Napoleon's military tactic in Mantua was to force their surrender by infecting the citizens with swamp fever.[68]
1835	Strychnine	Thomas Wainewright, who enjoyed the high society lifestyle, but was low on funds, had to resort to forging documents and taking out insurance policies on his victims with the aid of strychnine. Having worn out

		his welcome by poisoning his uncle and others, he fled to Tazmania and joined a chain gang.[69]
1855	Bubonic Plague	The Third Pandemic began in China and spread throughout all the continents. In China and India alone, 12 million people were killed due to this plague, which, until 1959, was still considered to be an active disease.[70]
1856	Strychnine	Dr. William Palmer was convicted of murdering his patient, John Parsons Cook, with strychnine. Dr. Palmer was only convicted of Cook's murder; but, he killed fifteen others: his wife, four of his children and his brother-in-law.[71]
1857	Arsenic	Madeleine Smith, daughter of a wealthy family in Glasgow, murdered her lover, Emile L'Angelier by the use of arsenic. She was released with a verdict of *not proven.*[72] The Arsenic Act of 1851 had already been in effect.
1860–1865	Biological Warfare	In his memoirs, W.T. Sherman gives an account of Confederate soldiers resorting to biological warfare by poisoning ponds with carcasses of dead animals.[73]
1871	Arsenic	C.F. Hall was an Arctic explorer who died under suspicious circumstances on his ship, Polaris. He and his crew were trying to discover the North Pole when Hall went into a coma and died. His death has been debated to have been either an accidental ingestion of arsenic or a deliberate murder.[74]
1876	Arsenic	Mary Stannard of New Haven County was murdered by her lover, Reverend H. H. Hayden, through an injection of arsenic; followed by him clubbing her and slitting her throat. Mary had, incorrectly, told Hayden that she was pregnant. Although enough evidence existed to convict him, the Jury (considering Hayden's social status) gave a verdict of not guilty and acquitted him. They believed his social status in the community shielded him from being found guilty.[75]
1910	Hyosine	Dr. Harvey Crippen was hanged for the alleged murder of his wife with the toxic hyosine. He was found guilty and hanged, although he maintained he was innocent.[76]

Date	Murder weapon	Event
1911	Arsenic	Fredrick Seddon poisoned his tenant for money using fly-paper which was soaked in arsenic, and administering it to his victim.[77]
1915	Anthrax	Dr. Anton Dilger, a German-American, grew cultures of Bacillus anthracis and Pseudomonas mallei in his Washington, D.C. home which were given to him by the German government. Dockworkers in Baltimore, sympathetic to the German cause, were equipped with the toxic agents and inoculation devices. They were instructed to infect three thousand horses, mules, and cattle which were on their way to the allied troops in Europe.[78]
1918	Influenza A	The Spanish Flu was pandemic in nature, killing between 50 and 100 million people worldwide in only 18 months. It did not originate in Spain.[79]
1920's	Poison Gas	Winston Churchill orders the RAF to use poison gas against the Kurds and the Arabs in Iraq to stem off a national revolt against the invading British forces.[80] *In 1988, Saddam Hussein gassed 5,000 Kurds. The world condemned Saddam Hussein's actions.
1931	Cholera	The Japanese military officials were involved in an attempt to poison the League of Nations commission members with cholera-infected fruit (the League was investigating Japan's siege of Manchuria).[81]
1931–1938	Arsenic	Twenty murders were committed by the "Great Arsenic Murder Ring" in South Philadelphia. The case came to be known as "The Poison Widow Case." The victims were mostly male and insurance policies had been taken out on them. Twenty-four people were eventually indicted and found guilty.[82]
1936	Biological Warfare	Shiro Ishii, a Japanese physician and army officer, spearheads the establishment of Unit 731. A 150- building complex was built in Manchuria, and another one in Changchun, so as to carry out biological warfare experiments. Ishii carried out these experiments on Chinese soldiers and civilians.[83]
1940–1941	Biological Warfare	October 4: Japanese released the plague bacteria in Chuhsien, China causing the deaths of twenty-one people. October 29: The plague bacteria were dropped by the

Date	Murder weapon	Event
		Japanese planes at Ninpo, China. ninety-nine people died. November 28: Biological bombs were dropped at Chinhua, but no deaths were reported. January, 1941: An epidemic broke out nearby. It killed many people.[84]
1941	Anthrax	The British become involved in experimenting with anthrax by establishing a complex off the Scottish coast.[85]
1941–1943	Biological Warfare	United States established Camp Detrick in Frederick, Maryland so as to study and develop biological warfare agents. In 1943, Camp Detrick was fully functional. Mississippi was the site chosen for field testing.[86]
1940–1950's	Arsenic	Nannie Doss was accused of murdering many family members, including five husbands.[87]
1940	Lewisite	The Germans had developed an organic gas from arsenic called Lewisite. Upon contact, the skin reacted by the appearance of huge blisters. The British response was to make an antidote to this agent and called it BAL (British Anti-Lewisite).[88]
1943–1945	Phenol (Carbolic acid)	Mengele, the notorious Nazi doctor arrived at Auschwitz in 1943. To make the camp more efficient as a killing apparatus, Mengele taught the other doctors to inject phenol into prisoners as they were standing in line. At first, they administered these injections in the arm, and eventually, to save time, the injections were given straight into the hearts of the victims. Mengele also injected poisons into living children so as to observe their reactions. He preferred experimenting on twins and dwarfs.[89]
1944	Cyanide	On October 14, two of Rommel's generals arrived at his home carrying a letter written by Hitler. In the letter, Hitler had instructed Rommel to kill himself in exchange for full military honors, as Rommel had been implicated in a plot to kill Hitler. Rommel took a cyanide pill and, twenty minutes later, his death was confirmed as he was driven away from his house.[90]
1945	Cyanide	Joseph Goebbels (the man behind the propaganda to exterminate Jews), realizing that Germany had lost the war, instructed an

Date	Murder weapon	Event
		SS doctor to inject his six children with morphine first so as to put them to sleep; then, they were given a lethal injection of cyanide. He and his wife were then shot to death.[91]
1945	Cyanide	Eva Braun, Hitler's mistress and newly wed, committed suicide by taking a cyanide pill a day after she and Hitler were married.[92] *Hitler did not take poison; he shot himself and then had asked that his body be burned.
1945	Cyanide	Himmler (head of the SS and the Gestapo) committed suicide by ingesting a cyanide pill while being given a medical exam by a British military doctor. Himmler could not believe that Germany had failed in her quest for world domination.[93]
1945	Barium Carbonate (rat poison)	The British army, stationed in Persia, were accidentally poisoned by pastry made of flour tainted with barium carbonate. No deaths were reported.[94]
1946	Arsenic	After the war, German soldiers were imprisoned in a German prison camp, Stalag 13, awaiting the results of the war trials set in motion by the Allies. Almost all of the Jews in a ghetto in Vilna, Lithuania had been exterminated. Those who survived devised a plan by painting three thousand loaves of bread, destined to be shipped to Stalag 13, with an arsenic solution obtained from French chemists. It has been suggested that 2,283 Germans died in this act of revenge.[95]
1954	Spanish Fly (Cantharidin)	Famous case in United Kingdom, where Arthur Ford is sent to prison for six years for inserting cantharidin in coconut candies, and offering them to his female colleagues who had spurned him earlier (he was married). His motive was to entice them, since he believed the myth that cantharidin was an aphrodisiac. Unfortunately, both women died. *Cantharidin was used by Marquis de Sade (1740–1814) to poison five prostitutes. De Sade believed in its aphrodisiac properties.[96]
1954	Cyanide	Alan Turing, English mathematician, who introduced the turing machine, laid the foundation for research in artificial intelligence; he helped in breaking the Enigma Code during World War II that the

Date	Murder weapon	Event
		Germans used for radio communications. Turing was found guilty of being a homosexual (a crime) and sentenced to estrogen treatments. He died of cyanide poisoning in an apparent suicide.[97]
1956	Arsenic	U.S. Ambassador to Italy, Clare Boothe Luce, became ill and had to resign from her post. The culprit was a ceiling in her bedroom which was fabricated out of arsenic-laden materials. The washing-machine on the upper floor, directly above the bedroom, caused vibrations and dislodged the arsenate as dust. The Ambassador and her husband, since the incident, were nicknamed, "Arsenic and Old Luce."[98]
1960's	Biological Warfare	Fecally-contaminated spear traps were utilized by the Vietcong during the Vietnam war.[99]
1963	Barium Chloride	In Israel, 100 people were poisoned accidentally after eating sausages made in Turkey. At first, the symptoms guided the doctors to declare food poisoning, but they soon realized none of the victims showed double vision and/or drooping of the eyelids. After analyzing the potassium levels in the blood (low in barium chloride poisoning), they found the source.[100]
1965–1966	Curare	Dr. Mario Jascalevich (Dr. X) was indicted in the killing of five hospital patients by administering lethal doses of curare. He wanted to discredit other doctors who had challenged his authority as chief surgeon. He was found not guilty in 1978.[101]
1970	Biological Warfare	A group (the Weathermen) that was opposed to the role of America in the Vietnam War, attempted to buy biological agents so as to contaminate the water supply in U.S. metropolitan areas.[102]
1972	Typhoid	Chicago was the location for the arrest of the right-wing organization "Order of the Rising Sun." They had in their possession 30–40 kg of typhoid cultures that they were about to use to poison the water supply in Chicago, St. Louis, and other Midwest cities.[103]
1972	Thallium	Thallium (pest control) was used by Graham Young in experiments conducted on family,

Date	Murder weapon	Event
		friends, and colleagues. The method of poisoning was mixing his poison with tea. He was sentenced to life in prison.[104]
1974	Cyanide	Ronald O'Brien spiked his own child's sherbet powder with cyanide, so as to claim an insurance policy he had taken out on his child's life. He was sentenced to prison.[105]
1975–1983	Yellow Rain	Planes and helicopters drop a multicolored aerosol known as the Yellow Rain on Laos and Kampuchea. It results in the deaths of both man and animals.[106]
1975	Arsenic	In Singapore, arsenic poisoning was found in seventy-four patients. The source was an array of antiasthmatic herbal preparations. High levels of arsenic have also been found in Chinese herbal balls sold in the Unmited States.[107]
1978	Cyanide	One of the largest mass suicides took place in Jonestown, Guyana. Led by Jim Jones, he and 913 members of his church (Peoples Temple) drank a cup of Flavor Aid laced with potassium cyanide.[108]
1978	Ricin	Georgi Markov, a Bulgarian dissident, was assassinated by the Soviet-controlled Bulgarian government. In London, as he was taking a walk on Waterloo Bridge, a specially equipped umbrella was utilized to inject a pellet coated with 450 micrograms of ricin into his leg. He died by the third day after suffering from nausea, tachycardia, fever, and bloody vomit. Cardiac arrest soon followed.[109]
1979	Anthrax	An accidental anthrax incident in the city of Sverdlovsk, U.S.S.R., led to the deaths of approximately one thousand people. The government at first denied the accident.[110]
1981	Anthrax	The "Dark Harvest Commandos" (environmental group) left packages of soil laced with anthrax outside a weapons research facility and a political party conference in Great Britain. Their motive was to bring attention to the contaminated soil on Gruinard Island.[111]
1982	Cyanide	The pain reliever Tylenol® was contaminated with cyanide causing the deaths of seven people in Chicago. Although the perpetrator was never found, James Lewis was arrested for attempting to extort

Date	Murder weapon	Event
		one million dollars from Johnson & Johnson after the incident. He was paroled in 1995.[112]
1984	Salmonella	An Indian religious cult, the Rajneesh, aimed to alter the outcome of a local election by contaminating salad bars in restaurants in Dalles and Wasco counties in Oregon using Salmonella typhimurium. Over 750 people were poisoned and 40 were hospitalized.[113]
1986	Cyanide	Stella Nickell of Washington tried poisoning her husband (Bruce Nickell) with various toxins and then attempted a coverup by murdering a random victim through lacing the OTC pain reliever, Excedrin, with cyanide. Bruce died on June 5th and the random stranger, Sue Snow, died on June 11th. Nickell was sentenced to ninety years in prison.[114]
1987	Pesticide	Pesticide was utilized to poison the water at a constabulary in Zamboanga City, Philippines. There were 19 fatalities and 140 injured.[115]
1987	Arsenic, Cyanide, Cleansers	Donald Harvey was responsible for the murders of of at least thirty-seven people, although he confessed that the number of his victims was closer to seventy people. He received eight life terms.[116]
1988–2004	Digoxin and Insulin	Charles Cullen confessed to killing forty patients over sixteen years working at different hospitals. His favorite poisons were digoxin (heart medicine) and insulin (diabetes medicine), both in high doses. He was sentenced to eighteen life sentences in prison.[117]
1989	Pavulon and Anectine	The Long Island's "Angel of Death" (Richard Angelo) killed his patients by injecting Pavulon and Anectine, (both paralyzing drugs) into the I.V. bags of unsuspecting patients, he created an emergency situation where he in turn could save them. He was sentenced to sixty-one years to life.[118]
1991	Cyanide	Joseph Meling, using cyanide-laced Sudafed capsules, tried to kill his wife so that he could collect on a $700,000 insurance policy. He tampered with other packages so as to divert attention. His wife, Jennifer, survived. Two other victims from Washington died.[119]

Date	Murder weapon	Event
1994	Chemical Warfare	Chemical grenades were used to attack a village in Ormancik, Turkey resulting in sixteen fatalities.[120]
1994	Chemical Warfare	Nerve gas attack in Matsumoto, Japan. It resulted in 7 deaths, and 270 people were injured.[121]
1995	Chemical Warfare	Shoko Asahara, the leader of the Japanese cult group, AUM Shinrikyo (Supreme Truth) and his followers released sarin gas in the subways of Tokyo, Japan. Five simultaneous attacks were coordinated and carried out. The attacks killed 12 and injured 5511 people.[122]
1995	Chemical Warfare	A month after the sarin attacks in Tokyo, tear gas was the weapon used in an attack in Yokohama, Japan. There were no fatalities, but 272 people were injured.[123]
1995	Yersinia pestis	Larry Wayne Harris, a laboratory technician from Ohio, ordered three vials of the plague bacterium (Yersinia pestis) using his credit card and a false letterhead. It was discovered that he was a member of a white supremacist organization. He could only be convicted of mail fraud. Laws prohibiting the sale of biological and chemical materials did not exist at the time of the conviction. These laws have since changed. These types of products can't be sold to individuals.[124]
1996	Shigella dysenteriae Type 2	In the tea room of a medical centre, muffins and doughnuts were intentionally contaminated with Shigella dysenteriae Type 2. This led to a major gastrointestinal illness in a dozen employees.[125]
1996	Insulin	"Martha U" was convicted of killing four geriatric patients, but was suspected of nine murders. None of the victims were terminally ill.[126]
1997	Arsenic and Potassium Injections	By the time of his conviction in 1997, Dr. Michael Swango had murdered sixty people using arsenic and potassium injections at various hospitals.[127]
1999	HIV	In the province of Nakhon Nayok in China, a widow whose husband had died of the AIDS, attempted to infect twenty policemen and several politicians with HIV.[128]
1999	HIV	In Zadar, Croatia, a criminal attempted to rob a currency exchange office by

Date	Murder weapon	Event
		threatening the employees with a syringe allegedly containing HIV.[129]
1999	Medical Waste	On August 17 and 19, two bags of medical wastes were found outside of two synagogues in Stamford and Norwalk, Connecticut.[130]
1999	Biological Warfare	Russian soldiers stumbled upon plans devised to use biological weapons on the bodies of dead Chechens killed during the fighting that took place in Dagestan.[131]
1999	Epinephrine and Potassium Chloride	Orville Lynn Majors, a nurse living in Clinton, Indiana, is convicted of six counts of murder. His killing spree began in 1993 and ended when he received life imprisonment in 1999. He had used a combination of epinephrine and potassium chloride. This mixture causes the work of the heart to rise and the blood pressure to spike before cardiac arrest occurs. It was suspected that Majors was involved in the deaths of 130 patients.[131]
2000	Morphine	Dr. Harold Shipman, convicted for the deaths of 15 patients, was given 15 life sentences. The authorities believe he might have murdered, more likely, close to 200 patients by using morphine as a poison. He utilized morphine as it causes CNS depression, leading to death within a short span of time. The onset of death can then be attributed to cardiac arrest or old age. He was finally caught when he falsified the will of one of his patients so inadequately that it roused the suspicion of the authorities. During the trial, he stated he used derogatory nicknames for his patients. One nickname: WOW-Whining Old Woman.[132]
2000	Midazolam	Surrey, England was the locale where Kevin Cobb, 38-year-old nurse, was convicted of murder, rape, and intent to rape. He injected his victims with midazolam, which is a sedative rendering short-term memory loss, and it can not be detected in the body after eight hours. After slipping the sedative into a fellow nurse, Susan Annis's cider, Cobb, wanted to rape her. Due to a heart problem, she instead died. Cobb received seven life

Date	Murder weapon	Event
		sentences for the murder and the other rapes he committed.[133]
2001	Anthrax	September 18: An assistant to the NBC news anchorman, Tom Brokaw, opens a letter laced with anthrax. Skin lesions, swelling, erythema soon develop, along with headache and black eschar. She recovers with antibiotics (diagnosis: Cutaneous anthrax). September 28: Seven-month-old son of an ABC producer is exposed to Cutaneous anthrax at his mother's workplace. He recovers. October 2: Robert Stevens and his coworker, Ernest Blanco, are exposed to inhalation anthrax. Blanco recovers, but Stevens dies.
2001	Anthrax	October 14: An aide to Senate Majority Leader, Tom Daschle, opens a letter tainted with anthrax. Capitol Hill is contaminated and twenty-eight personnel are exposed. October 21, 22: Two postal workers handling mail at the post office center which had received the letter to Tom Daschle's office, died of inhalation anthrax. October 25: 10,000 people were estimated to have been placed on prophylactic antibiotics (Cipro). October 28: Kathy Nguyen, working at the Manhattan Eye, Ear, and Throat Hospital became ill; she wasdiagnosed with inhalation anthrax, and died three days later. November 2: CDC confirmed six cases of cutaneous Anthrax and ten cases of inhalation anthrax (2-FL, 1 NJ 2-NJ, 5-Washington, D.C.). Five cases were suspected of being anthrax.[134]
2001	Pavulon	Efren Saldivar admitted to killing from sixty to hundred patients using the poison, Pavulon. This is a synthetic paralytic, imitating the effects of curare. In high doses, it causes paralysis of the muscles, and the lungs stop functioning, but the victim can't signal for help. Saldivar is serving a life sentence.[135]
2001	Vecuronium	Daisuke Mori was arrested in Japan and charged with the murder of an 89-year-old patient and attempted murder of three children and a 45-year-old man. Mori, a nurse, injected his victims with a muscle relaxant by changing the intravenous drip

Date	Murder weapon	Event
		bag prepared by others with one of his own containing the poison.[136]
2002	Mivacurium Chloride	Vickie Dawn Jackson of Texas was indicted in the murder of four patients at the hospital where she worked. She injected her victims with a muscle relaxant, stopping their breathing. She was indicted with 3three more counts of murder after ten bodies were exhumed. She was suspected to have participated in the killing of at least twenty-five patients.[137]
2002	Cyanide	A suicide bomber working for HAMAS detonated an explosive in Netanay, Israel killing twenty-nine Israelis. The IDF reported the suicide bomber was supposed to have cyanide attached to the belt-bomb, but the poison itself was unsuccessful.[138]
2002	Cyanide	Chechen rebels plotted to sell vodka tainted with a potassium cyanide solution at markets in Grozny.[139]
2002	Pesticide	At the Johanne Marange Apostolic Church in Zimbabwe, seven people died and forty-seven others became severely sick after drinking tea laced with poison. Authorities believed it was an intentional act.[140]
2002	Fentanyl Gas	The Russian government storms a theatre in Moscow to free 800 people held hostage by Chechen rebels. Fentanyl was the gas used to carry out the operation, resulting in the deaths of over 100 people with an additional 245 hospitalized. All of the Chechen rebels were killed when the assault occurred.[141]
2003	Arsenic	At the Adolph Luteran Church in New Sweden, Maine, one church member died and sixteen other members fell ill after drinking coffee which was laced with arsenic. Investigators believed the poisoning was deliberate.[142]
2003	Poisons	The Dutch nurse, Lucy Quirina de Berk, was indicted on eight counts of murder and attempted murder. The authorities suspected she might have been involved in more than thirty cases. The victims' ages were from six-month-old infant to a 91-year-old man. De Berk was a former prostitute who had lied about her degree and credentials. She was convicted of the murders of four

Date	Murder weapon	Event
		patients and given a life sentence. After her appeal in 2004, she received additional life in prison for seven murder charges.[143]
2004	Painkillers	Roger Andermatt, a Swiss nurse, killed twenty-two elderly patients at a nursing home in Lucerne, Switzerland. Over a period of six years, Andermatt utilized lethal injections of painkillers and/or suffocated patients with plastic bags. He was sentenced to life in prison.[144]
2006	Morphine and Versed	During the Hurricane Katrina, Dr. Anna Pou and two nurses, Cheri Landry and Lori Budo, utilized Versed and morphine to murder four patients at Memorial Medical Center, according to the Louisiana's attorney general. The doctor and the two nurses had denied any wrongdoing, arguing that due to the extreme conditions present, many of the patients died instead from dehydration. The coroner has declared the cause of deaths as to be "undetermined". The case is still pending.[145]
2007	Polonium-210	Alexander Litvinenko, a former Russian KGB spy, died after ingesting the radioactive isotope, Polonium-210. He lived in London, England.[146] His death was not the first one from the isotope. The first victim was Nobus Yamada, a Japanese researcher working in Marie Curie's lab in 1924 in France.[147]

APPENDIX B: DRUG-ATMS

TWO COMPANIES ARE RESHAPING THE WORLD OF PHARMACY

There is a revolution going on in Southern California, and it is spreading rapidly across America. Two companies, Asteres Incorporated in Del Mar and Distributed Delivery Networks Corporation (ddn) in San Marcos, own the market (and patents) on ATM-type machines that deliver refill medications to patients. The advocates and owners of the drug-ATMs say the machines free pharmacists to spend more time with customers. Opponents argue that the devices are substituting arguable convenience for safety—distancing patients from the pharmacist.

Between the two companies, these automated drug kiosks are popping up in pilot programs in Reston, VA (Asteres), Penn Station in New York City (ddn), and Longs Drugs Store in Del Mar (Asteres). Negotiations with pharmacy boards in several other states, including Ohio, Connecticut, Delaware, Illinois, Minnesota, Wisconsin, and Maryland, are underway to open up new test markets.

Asteres calls its machine the ScriptCenter; Distributed Delivery Networks Corporation calls its machine the Pharmaceutical Automated Product Machine, or APM. A ScriptCenter machine will cost between $65,000 and $95,000. A ddn machine ranges from $45,000 to $60,000, and ddn is reported to be working on a smaller contraption that would cost about $40,000. The two companies had been embroiled in litigation for months, both sides running up significant legal fees, but have settled their differences. Both sides have decided, instead, to carve up the national market. All indications are that both companies will become fantastically wealthy, and this new technology will spread like wildfire. Distributed's president, Bill Holmes, has been widely interviewed, including a piece on "Good Morning America" with Diane Sawyer and a reference on John Stewart's "The Daily Show." It appears that people are taking notice of this new technology.

As of May 2007, Holme's Distributed Delivery Networks Corporation had been formally and completely "acquired" by Parata Systems of Durham, North Carolina. Together with the recent acquisition of the assets of Amistar and the Automated Prescription Systems business of McKesson Corporation, Parata is positioned to become the leader in prescription "pick-up" kiosk technology. Parata was founded in 2001 to grow the safety and efficiency of the retail pharmacy sector. Distributed Delivery Network's core team has stayed on with Parata to support its customer base and work to increase regulatory acceptance in new markets nationwide.[1]

THE MACHINES

The drug-ATMs have multiple levels of built-in safeguards. There are personal customer codes that are linked to personal credit card identification; there are also bar-code scanners and passwords to insure that the drugs reach the right patient. To pick up a medication item, a customer must enter a PIN number on a touch screen and then swipe a credit card to receive a labeled and bagged product that drops from a chute. The companies, through multiple media interviews and press releases, promote their products as following in the tradition of conventional mail order pharmacies and drive-up windows. They claim the margin for error is virtually zero. In 2004, prescription drug sales by mail order accounted for 14 percent of the market—up from 10 percent in 1999. Longs Drugs in Del Mar reports that nearly 1,000 customers have already signed up at three different stores, accounting for over 10 percent of medication refills.

PHARMACISTS ARE ALARMED

Fred Mayer, president of Pharmacists Planning Service Inc. (PPSI), a nonprofit organization in San Rafael, California, has been quoted (in multiple sources) in vehement opposition to the drug-ATM concept. Pharmacy-OneSource (www.pharmacyonesource.com), an industry news site reveals that most pharmacists support Mayer's position. The site notes that nearly 68 percent of pharmacists polled were "strongly opposed" to the new technology, with another 12 percent counted as "opposed." The pharmacists believe that customers, particularly seniors, need the input and consultation of a live human being (even for refills) and argue that the potential for robbery and muggings is gravely underestimated. Pharmacists argue that, even for the average drug consumer, significant health risks exist when a doctorate-trained professional is replaced with a machine. A commonly cited example is the acne drug Accutane (isotretinoin, Hoffman-la Roche) that can pose serious health risks to women who are or may become pregnant.[2–4]

IMPLICATIONS FOR PHYSICIANS AND PATIENTS

With the American Medical Association (AMA) and many of its subspecialty members fighting multiple battles on multiple fronts to prevent dentists, podiatrists, chiropractors, nurse practitioners, and nurse anesthetists from encroaching on the traditional "scope of practice" of physicians, this seemingly unstoppable technological trend in pharmacy should be a cause for alarm. Once the rank of pharmacists (and the stature, number of qualified applicants to pharmacy schools, market incentives, etc.) is thinned by robotic replacements, how many doctors of pharmacy will be available to discuss and educate the increasing number of drugs being dispensed to an everaging population? How should a physician feel about writing a prescription with refills that will be dispensed by a drug-ATM? Where does the process end?

Are there any implications in the implementation of this technology that portend trouble in securing our pharmaceutical supply? The makers of these drug-ATMs will claim that their scanning and tracking software keep better tabs on medications. What they will not disclose is the fact that they are only scanning and recording the container, not the medication itself. By distancing themselves from their targets, terrorists could utilize these machines to disseminate more contaminated drugs to more people, and in a more efficient fashion.

Notes

Chapter 1

1. Eugene W. Hickok, 2004. Address of the U.S. Department of Education (the Deputy Secretary) on Jill St. Claire's Homeland Security U.S. Net website, "Threats to Schools." http://www.homelandsecurityus.net/America%20Threats/threats_to_schools. htm (accessed January 26, 2007).

2. Ibid.

3. Tamar Nordenberg, 2000. *FDA Consumer* Magazine. Make No Mistake: Medical Errors Can Be Deadly Serious. http://www.fda.gov/fdac/features/2000/500_err.html (accessed February 20, 2007).

Chapter 2

1. Lazo Brunton and Keith Parker, 2005. *Goodman and Gillman's The Pharmacological Basis of Therapeutics*, Ed. 11. New York: McGraw Hill Publishing.

2. The Cancer Cure Foundation, 2007. Medical Errors, The FDA, and Problems with Prescription Drugs. http://www.cancure.org/medical_errors.htm (accessed January 26, 2007).

3. World Health Organization, 2007. Counterfeit Medicines. http://www.who.int/mediacentre/factsheets/fs275/en (accessed January 13, 2007).

4. Second Annual San Diego Health Policy Conference, June 9, 2006. Terrorism, International Crime, and Medicine Security: Issues in a Global Marketplace. California Western School of Law. San Diego, CA.

5. Second Annual San Diego Health Policy Conference, June 9, 2006. Terrorism, International Crime, and Medicine Security: Issues in a Global Marketplace. California Western School of Law. San Diego, CA.

6. Institute of Medicine of the National Academies, 2007. Home page. http://www.iom.edu (accessed February 20, 2007).

Chapter 3

1. CNN.com, 2005. Gunmen Attack Iraq Hospital, Free Suspected Insurgent. http://www.cnn.com/2005/WORLD/meast/12/07/iraq.main/index.html (accessed January 28, 2007).

2. CNN.com, 2003. Official: Credible Threats Pushed Terror Alert Higher. http://www.cnn.com/2003/US/02/07/threat.level/index.html (accessed January 28, 2007).

3. Comic Convention, June 2006, San Diego Convention Center. Interview with Cast and Crew of the film *Snakes on a Plane* for snakesonablog.com.

4. *New York Times*, December 16, 2003. Health Care Workers Who Kill. NY Region.

5. Pyrek, Kelly, 2006. Healthcare Serial Killers: Recognizing the Red Flags. *Forensic Nurse.* http://www.forensicnursemag.com/articles/391feat1.html (accessed August 29, 2006).

6. Associated Press, October 6, 2006. Nurse Gets Life Term in 10 Patients' Deaths. *The San Diego Union-Tribune.* http://sharpnet/news/display.cfm?ID=16999 (accessed October 6, 2006).

7. *California Healthline*, California HealthCare Foundation, 2005. DHS Letter States Hospitals Are Not Specific Targets of Terrorist Attack. June 10. The Advisory Board Company. http://r01.webmail.aol.com/20221/aol/en-us/mail/display-message.aspx (accessed October 6, 2006).

8. Institute of Medicine of the National Academies, 2007. Home page. http://www.iom.edu (accessed February 20, 2007).

Chapter 4

1. Second Annual San Diego Health Policy Conference, June 9, 2006. Terrorism, International Crime, and Medicine Security: Issues in a Global Marketplace. California Western School of Law, San Diego, CA.

2. Ibid.

3. Ibid.

4. Ibid.

5. World Health Organization, 2007. Review of IMPACT and Other Initiatives. http://www.who.int/hia/en (accessed January 25, 2007).

6. Ibid.

7. *New Scientist*, 2007. Review of Niger 1995 fake vaccine incident. http://www.newscientist.com/channel/health/mg19125683.900-the-medicines-that-could-kill-millions.html (accessed January 25, 2007).

8. Center for Medicine in the Public Interest, 2006. Counterfeit Drugs and China. http://www.cmpi.org/newsDetail.asp?contentdetailid=67&contenttypeid=3 (accessed December 21, 2006).

9. Ibid.

10. *Medical News Today*, 2007. Life Scan Blood Glucose Test Strips Counterfeit Warning, Canada. http://www.medicalnewstoday.com/medicalnews.php?newsid=55115 (accessed January 25, 2007).

11. Ibid.

12. Second Annual San Diego Health Policy Conference, June 9, 2006. Terrorism, International Crime, and Medicine Security: Issues in a Global Marketplace. California Western School of Law, San Diego, CA.

13. Ibid.

14. Ibid.

15. Ibid.

16. Ibid.

17. Ibid.

18. Ibid.

19. U.S. Food and Drug Administration, 2005. http://www.fda.gov/oc/initiatives/counterfeit/update2005.html (accessed September 11, 2006).

20. Greising, David and Bruce Japson, November 20, 2005. Pharmaceutical Companies Feeling Potent Effect of Fakes. *Chicago Tribune.*

21. U.S. Food and Drug Administration, 2005. http://www.fda.gov/oc/initiatives/counterfeit/update2005.html (accessed September 11, 2006).

22. Patient Care Technology Systems, 2007. Leading Hospitals Nationwide Select Automatic Tracking Solutions from Patient Care Technology System. http://www.pcts.com/News?Press/press_010907.asp (accessed January 17, 2007).

23. Ibid.

24. Doctor Click/Circling the Dome: Technology has Unleashed Torrents of Possibilities for Saving Lives. *Hopkins Medicine,* Winter 2007, 30(2).

25. Ibid.

26. Donald G. McNeil Jr., 2007. *New York Times.* In the World of Life-Saving Fakes, A Growing Epidemic of Deadly Fakes. http://www.nytimes.com/2007/02/20/science/20coun.html?_r=2&oref=slogin&ref=health&pagewanted=all&oref=slogin (accessed February 20, 2007).

27. Ibid.

28. Ibid.

29. Agency for Healthcare Research and Quality, 2007. Medical Errors: The Scope of the Problem. http://www.ahrq.gov/qual/errback.htm (accessed February 19, 2007).

Chapter 5

1. David Brown, April 22, 2005. Fake Hospital Inspectors Probed (FBI Investigates Incidents at Facilities in Boston, Detroit, LA). *Washington Post,* A10.

2. Ibid.

3. Ibid.

4. John Andrew, May 2003. It's Always "Orange Alert" for Health Facility Security—News on the Cover. *Healthcare Purchasing News.* http://findarticles.com/p/articles/mi_m0BPC/is_5_27/ai_101797120 (accessed November 3, 2006).

5. Ibid.

6. Ibid.

7. Securityinfo Watch, July 18, 2006. Fighting Intrusion of Violence into Hospitals. Securityinfo Watch website (*The Baltimore Sun* via NewsEdge Corporation). http://www.simon-net.com/online/Healthcare-Facilities/Fighting-Intrusion-of-Violence-into-Hospitals@HealthcareFacilities (accessed November 3, 2006).

8. University of Kentucky, 2003. University of Kentucky Safety and Security Measures. http://www.uky.edu/PR/News/Archives/2003/March2003/03-03_safety_security.htm (accessed February 10, 2007).

9. University of Kentucky, 2002. *University of Kentucky News.* http://www.uky.edu/PR/UK_News/news80502.html (accessed February 10, 2007).

10. Institute of Medicine of the National Academies, 2006. June Report Brief: The Future of Emergency Care in the United States Health System. National Academies Press of the National Academy of Sciences, Washington, D.C. http://www.nap.edu (accessed January 28, 2007).

11. Ibid.

12. Ibid.

13. Susan Lewis, 2007. *NOVA Online*—History of Biowarfare. http://www.pbs.org/wgbh/nova/bioterror/history.html (accessed February 10, 2007).

14. Michael Phillips, 2005.BioTerrorism: A Brief History. *Northeast Florida Medicine.* http://www.dcmsonline.org/jaxmedicine/2005journals/bioterrorism/bioterrorism_history (accessed February 10, 2007).

15. Securityinfo Watch, July 18, 2006. Fighting Intrusion of Violence into Hospitals. Securityinfo Watch website (*The Baltimore Sun* via NewsEdge Corporation). http://www.simon-net.com/online/Healthcare-Facilities/Fighting-Intrusion-of-Violence-into-Hospitals@HealthcareFacilities (accessed November 3, 2006).

16. John Andrew, 2003. It's Always "Orange Alert" for Health Facility Security—News on the Cover. *Healthcare Purchasing News.* http://findarticles.com/p/articles/mi_m0BPC/is_5_27/ai_101797120 (accessed February 10, 2007).

17. KARE 11, January 26, 2006. Man Charged with Raping Woman at Hospital. KARE 11 website. http://www.kare11.com/news/news_article.aspx?storyid=117235 (accessed November 3, 2006).

18. WRAL, September 1, 2006. Hospital Increases Security After Gang Threat. WRAL website. http://www.wral.com/news/9780534/detail.html (accessed November 3, 2006).

19. WDBJ 7, August 28, 2006. Hospitals Review Security Procedures After Shooting. WDBJ 7 website. http://www.wdbj7.com/Global/story.asp?S=5336686&nav=S6ak (accessed November 3, 2006).

20. Securityinfo Watch, July 18, 2006. Fighting Intrusion of Violence into Hospitals. Securityinfo Watch website (*The Baltimore Sun* via NewsEdge Corporation). http://www.simon-net.com/online/Healthcare-Facilities/Fighting-Intrusion-of-Violence-into-Hospitals@HealthcareFacilities (accessed November 3, 2006).

21. Hannah Baldwin, May 30, 2006. Hospitals are Vulnerable to Terrorist Attack, Claim University Experts. Loughborough University Public Relations Office website http://r01.webmail.aol.com/20221/aol/en-us/mail/display-message.aspx (accessed October 4, 2006).

22. Dan Hanfling, July 18, 2002. Preparedness: Hospital Readiness. *Washington Post* Live Online Discussion. http://www.washingtonpost.com.nation_hanfling071802.html (accessed October 4, 2006).

23. George Stungis and Thomas Schori, March 2003. A Terrorist Target Selection and Prioritization Model, *Journal of Homeland Security.*

24. Adam Dorin, 2006. Anatomy of a Public Health Crisis, Terrorism: Should ASCs Take an Active Role in Homeland Defense? *SAMBA Newsletter,* 21(3): 9–11. Excerpts from author's own work, with permission. http://www.sambahq.org/professional-info/newsletter/July2006.pdf (accessed February 4, 2007).

25. Official U.S. Government Booklet, *Survival Under Atomic Attack,* 1950. Distributed and Reprinted by the Office of Civil Defense, State of California, Under Governor Earl Warren. Executive Office of the President, National Security Resources Board; Civil Defense Office. California State Printing Division. NSRB Doc. 130.

26. Adam Dorin, 2006. Anatomy of a Public Health Crisis, Terrorism: Should ASCs Take an Active Role in Homeland Defense? *SAMBA Newsletter,* 21(3): 9–11. Excerpts from author's own work, with permission. http://www.sambahq.org/professional-info/newsletter/July2006.pdf (accessed February 4, 2007).

27. Ibid.

28. The White House, 2004. Project BioShield: Progress in the War on Terror.http://www.whitehouse.gov/infocus/bioshield (accessed February 14, 2007).

29. Mike Mitka, February 14, 2007. Bioterror Vaccine Production: Take 2 (New Biodefense R&D Agency Created), *Journal of the American Medical Association,* 297(6).

30. U.S. Senator Richard Burr, 2007. Senator Richard Burr Introduces Comprehensive Biodefense Legislation. http://burr.senate.gov/index.cfm?FuseAction=Press Releases.Detail&PressRelease_id=121&Month=10&Year=2005 (accessed February 14, 2007).

31. Mike Mitka, February 14, 2007. Bioterror Vaccine Production: Take 2 (New Biodefense R&D Agency Created), *Journal of the American Medical Association,* 297(6).

32. Adam Dorin, 2006. Anatomy of a Public Health Crisis, Terrorism: Should ASCs Take an Active Role in Homeland Defense? *SAMBA Newsletter,* 21(3): 9–11. Excerpts from author's own work, with permission. http://www.sambahq.org/professional-info/newsletter/July2006.pdf (accessed February 4, 2007).

33. Gary Null et al., 2007. The American Medical System is the Leading Cause of Death and Injury in the United States. http://www.ourcivilisation.com/medicine/usamed.htm (accessed February 18, 2007).

Chapter 6

1. Alison Sebastian, October 30, 2002. Johnson's Russia List: Russia Confirms Siege Gas Based on Fentanyl. http://www.cdi.org/russia/johnson/6523-1.cfm (accessed January 25, 2007).

2. Lois Ember, November 4, 2002. *Chemical and Engineering News,* Opiate Ends Hostage Crisis (Fentanyl Used to Incapacitate Chechens Likely Doesn't Violate Chemical Arms Ban). http://pubs.acs.org/ cen/topstory/8044/8044notw1.html (accessed January 29, 2007).

3. Y. Vidal, 2002. *Outcry,* 101 Ways to Prevent Medical Errors. http://www.101 waystopreventerrors.com/laboratory.htm (accessed February 10, 2007).

Chapter 7

1. FBI Report, August 18, 1997. Emergency Response & Research Institute, Excerpts: FBI Report on Domestic Terrorism, *ERRI Daily Intelligence Report,* 3:230.

2. JM Howell, M. Altieri, and J. Fletcher, Eds., 1998, *Emergency Medicine.* Philadelphia: WB Saunders & Co.

3. DM LaCombe, GT Miller, and JD Dennis, May 2004. Primary Blast Injury: An EMS Guide to Pathophysiology, Assessment, and Management. *JEMS,* 29(5): 70–72, 74, 76–78, 80–81, 86–89.

4. TW Sharp, RJ Brennan, M Keim, et al., Aug. 1998. Medical Preparedness for a Terrorist Incident Involving Chemical or Biological Agents During the 1996 Atlanta Olympic Games. *Ann. Emerg. Med.*; 32(2): 214–223.

5. JB Tucker, Aug. 6, 1997. National Health and Medical Services Response to Incidents of Chemical and Biological Terrorism, *JAMA,* 278(5): 362–368.

6. Emergent BioSolutions, 2007. Biopharmaceutical Company website. http://www.emergentbiosolutions.com (accessed February 18, 2007).

7. JG Breman, DA Henderson, 2002. Diagnosis and management of smallpox. *New England Journal of Medicine,* 346: 1300–1308.

8. Medical University of South Carolina, 2007. Travel Clinic website. http://www.muschealth.com/travelclinic/vaccines.htm (accessed February 18, 2007).

9. US Environmental Protection Agency, 2006. Guarding Against Terrorist and Security Threats (Suggested Measures for Drinking Water and Wastewater Utilities). http://www.waterisac.org (accessed December 7, 2006).

10. Mary Beth Sheridan, December 12, 2006. Study: Maryland and D.C. Not Prepared for Health Emergencies. http://www.washingtonpost.com/wp-dyn/content/article/2006/12/12/AR2006121200988 (accessed December 12, 2006).

11. *Medical News Today*, 2007. U.S. Medical Care is the Most Expensive and Has the Most Errors. http://www.medicalnewstoday.com/healthnews.php?newsid=33003 (accessed February 20, 2007).

Chapter 8

1. Newt Gingrich, November 27, 2006. Speech to the Nackey S. Loeb School of Communications—Gingrich Communications. http://www.newt.org/backpage.asp?art=38.19 (accessed January 3, 2007).

2. The JCAHO (Joint Commission on Accreditation of Healthcare Organizations), 2007. Website for Accreditation Standards. http://www.jointcommission.org (accessed January 14, 2007).

3. The AAAHC (Accreditation Association for Ambulatory Health Care), 2007. Website for Accreditation Standards. http://www.aaahc.org (accessed January 14, 2007).

4. The AAAASF (American Association for Accreditation of Ambulatory Surgery Facilities, Inc.), 2007. Website for Accreditation Standards. http://www.aaaasf.org (accessed January 20, 2007).

5. The NFPA (National Fire Protection Association), 2007. Website for Fire Safety Standards, including the NFPA Life Safety Code 101-2000 and NFPA 99: Health Care Facilities. http://www.nfpa.org (accessed January 20, 2007).

6. Occupational Safety and Health Administration (OSHA), 2007. Website for Statutes, Standards, and Protocols. http://www.osha.gov (accessed January 20, 2007).

7. The JCAHO (Joint Commission on Accreditation of Healthcare Organizations), 2007. Website for Accreditation Standards. http://www.jointcommission.org (accessed January 14, 2007).

8. Elizabeth Weise, 2005. *USA Today*, Medical Errors Still Claiming Many Lives. *http://www.usatoday.com/news/health/2005-05-17-medical-errors_x.htm* (accessed February 16, 2007).

Chapter 9

1. Michelle Meadows, 2004. *FDA Consumer* Magazine: The FDA and the Fight Against Terrorism. http://www.fda.gov/FDAC/features/2004/104_terror.html (accessed January 30, 2007).

2. Ibid.

3. U.S. Department of Health and Human Services, 2007. Summary of the HIPAA Privacy Rule. http://www.hhs.gov/ocr/privacysummary.pdf (accessed February 2, 2007).

4. Jeffrey L Arnold, 2002. Disaster Medicine in the 21st Century: Future Hazards, Vulnerabilities, and Risk. *Prehospital and Disaster Medicine* 17(1): 8.

5. John Marke, 2007. *A Legal/Regulatory Context for Managing Global Risk* (Draft Copy, Ver. 1.5 and personal communication: Deloitte-Touche, LLP, Washington, D.C.).

6. Ibid.

7. Ibid.

8. Y.Y. Haimes, 2004. *Risk Modeling, Assessment, and Management*, Second Edition. New York: Wiley & Sons.

9. National Research Council, 2002. *Preparing for the Revolution: Information Technology and the Future of the Research University*. Washington, D.C.: The National Academies Press.

10. Tamar Nordenberg, 2000. *FDA Consumer* Magazine. Make No Mistake: Medical Errors Can Be Deadly Serious. http://www.fda.gov/fdac/features/2000/500_err.html (accessed February 20, 2007).

Chapter 10

1. Joel W. McMaster, 2006. Chapter Seven: PK beyond cosmetic surgery—Uses of PK MAC for Mass Casualty Situations. In: *Anesthesia in Cosmetic Surgery—Minimally Invasive Anesthesia for Minimally Invasive Surgery* (Ed. Barry L. Friedberg, M.D., draft, prepublication by permission of the editor). New York: Cambridge University Press.

2. Nancy Solomon, 2003. Saint Louis University NewsLink. Enlisting Nurses in the War on Terrorism. http://www.slu.edu/readstory/newslink/2238 (accessed February 10, 2007).

3. Institute for BioSecurity, 2007. Saint Louis University School of Public Health website. http://www.bioterrorism.slu.edu/radiological.htm (accessed February 10, 2007).

4. Mershon Center for International Securities Study, 2006. The Ohio State University: Terror's Fourth Wave. http://mershoncenter.osu.edu/expertise/force/terror.htm (accessed February 10, 2007).

5. Ibid.

6. L Kohn, J Corrigan, and M Donaldson, 1999. *To Err is Human: building a safer health system.* Washington, D.C.: National Academy Press.7. *Science Daily*, 2004. U.S. Food and Drug Administration. FDA Announces New Initiative to Protect the U.S. Drug Supply Through the Use of Radiofrequency Identification Technology. http://www.sciencedaily.com/releases/2004/11/041124160812.htm (accessed February 13, 2007).

8. Ibid.

9. Ibid.

10. AdvaMed., 2003. Advanced Medical Technology Association. Government Reform Committee, Hearing on Project BioShield: Contracting for the Health and Security of the American Public. http://www.advamed.org/publicdocs/gr_bioshield_stmt.pdf (accessed February 14, 2007).

11. Ibid.

12. Ibid.

13. Paul Frenzen, 2007. CDC: Emerging Infectious Diseases. http://www.cdc.gov/ncidod/EID/vol10no9/03-0403.htm (accessed February 20, 2007).

Chapter 11

1. Adam Dorin, May 2007. Pushing the Envelope in Office-Based Anesthesia (Safe Surgery and Safe Anesthesia in the Office Setting). Presentation to the Society of Ambulatory Anesthesia (SAMBA). SAMBA Annual Meeting, San Diego.

2. Ibid.

3. Linda Aiken et al., 2002. *JAMA*. Hospital Nurse Staffing and Patient Mortality, Nurse Burnout and Job Dissatisfaction. http://jama.ama-assn.org/cgi/content/abstract/288/16/1987 (accessed February 21, 2007).

4. BE Landon, 2006. Quality of Care for the Treatment of Acute Medical Conditions in U.S. Hospitals. *Archives of Internal Medicine* 166: 2511–2517.

Chapter 12

1. Al. Heller, February 2007. Technology, Culture Foster Anesthesia-Pharmacy Teamwork. *Clinical Anesthesiology*, 35.

2. Ibid.

3. Docusys, 2007. Docusys with Docucart O.R. Series: The First Integrated Medication and Anesthesia Information System for the O.R. http://www.docusys.net/docs/DocuSys_DocuCart_OR_Series_Brochure.pdf (accessed February 17, 2007).

4. Picis, 2007. Picis is the Only Software Solution for High Acuity Care. http://www.picis.com (accessed February 17, 2007).

5. U.S. Department of Homeland Security, March 2007. Soft Targets Awareness Course, Williamsburg, Virginia. http://www.iaam.org/2004_meetings/dhs/DHS%20Soft%20Target%20Awareness%20Course%20for%20Jamestown,%20VA%20March%206-9,%202007.pdf (accessed February 20, 2007).

Appendix A

1. CBWInfo, 2005. A Brief History of Chemical, Biological, and Radiological Weapons—Ancient Times to the 19th Century. http://www.cbwinfo.com/History/ancto19th.shtml (accessed February 17, 2007).

2. JH Trestrail, 2000. *Criminal Poisoning: Investigational Guide for Law Enforcement, Toxicologists, Forensic Scientists, and Attorneys*, Totowa, NJ: Humana Press.

3. Anil Aggrawal, 1997. The Poison Sleuths. Poisons, Antidotes, and Anecdotes. http://www.tripos.com/~Prof_Anil_Aggrawal/poiso001.html (accessed February 11, 2007).

4. JH Trestrail, 2000. *Criminal Poisoning: Investigational Guide for Law Enforcement, Toxicologists, Forensic Scientists, and Attorneys.*, Totowa, NJ: Humana Press.

5. Anil Aggrawal, 1997. The Poison Sleuths. Poisons, Antidotes, and Anecdotes. http://www.tripos.com/~Prof_Anil_Aggrawal/poiso001.html (accessed February 11, 2007).

6. Gunnora Hallakarva, 1994. The Silent Weapon—Poisons and Antidotes in the Middle Ages. http://www.Gunnora.Hallakarva@f555.n387.zl.fidonet.org (accessed February 18, 2007).

7. Ibid.

8. Anil Aggrawal, 1997. The Poison Sleuths. Poisons, Antidotes, and Anecdotes. http://www.tripos.com/~Prof_Anil_Aggrawal/poiso001.html (accessed February 11, 2007).

9. Bio-Terry, 2007. History of Bioterrorism. A Chronological History of Bioterrorism and Biowarfare Throughout the Ages. http://www.bioterry.com/HistoryBioTerr.html. (accessed February 16, 2007).

10. Ibid.

11. CBWInfo, 2005. A Brief History of Chemical, Biological, and Radiological Weapons—Ancient Times to the 19th Century. http://www.cbwinfo.com/History/ancto19th.shtml (accessed February 17, 2007).

12. Ibid.

13. JH Trestrail, 2000. *Criminal Poisoning: Investigational Guide for Law Enforcement, Toxicologists, Forensic Scientists, and Attorneys.* Totowa, NJ: Humana Press.

14. Ibid.

15. CBWInfo, 2005. A Brief History of Chemical, Biological, and Radiological Weapons—Ancient Times to the 19th Century. http://www.cbwinfo.com/History/ancto19th.shtml (accessed February 17, 2007).

16. JH Trestrail, 2000. *Criminal Poisoning: Investigational Guide for Law Enforcement, Toxicologists, Forensic Scientists, and Attorneys,* Totowa, NJ: Humana Press.

17. JH Trestrail, 2000. *Criminal Poisoning: Investigational Guide for Law Enforcement, Toxicologists, Forensic Scientists, and Attorneys,* Totowa, NJ: Humana Press.

18. P. Retief Francois and Louise Cilliers, 2007. Poisons, Poisoning, and Poisoners in Rome. http://www.medicinaantiqua.org.uk/Medant/poisons.htm (accessed February 11, 2007).

19. Ibid.

20. Technology Museum of Thessaloniki, 2001. Ancient Greek Scientists. http://www.tmth.edu.gr/en/aet/12/70.html (accessed February 20, 2007).

21. Bio-Terry, 2007. History of Bioterrorism. A Chronological History of Bioterrorism and Biowarfare Throughout the Ages. http://www.bioterry.com/HistoryBioTerr.html. (accessed February 16, 2007).

22. The National Great Blacks in Wax Museum, 2007. Hannibal. http://ngbiwm.com/Exhibits/Hannibal.htm (accessed February 19, 2007).

23. CBWInfo, 2005. A Brief History of Chemical, Biological, and Radiological Weapons—Ancient Times to the 19th Century. http://www.cbwinfo.com/History/ancto19th.shtml (accessed February 17, 2007).

24. JH Trestrail, 2000. *Criminal Poisoning: Investigational Guide for Law Enforcement, Toxicologists, Forensic Scientists, and Attorneys,* Totowa, NJ: Humana Press.

25. WJ Meek, 1955. The gentle art of poisoning, *Journal of the American Medical Association,* 158:335–339.

26. CBWInfo, 2005. A Brief History of Chemical, Biological, and Radiological Weapons—Ancient Times to the 19th Century. http://www.cbwinfo.com/History/ancto19th.shtml (accessed February 17, 2007).

27. Gunnora Hallakarva, 1994. The Silent Weapon—Poisons and Antidotes in the Middle Ages. http://www.Gunnora.Hallakarva@f555.n387.zl.fidonet.org (accessed February 18, 2007).

28. Ibid.

29. Gunnora Hallakarva, 1994. The Silent Weapon—Poisons and Antidotes in the Middle Ages. http://www.Gunnora.Hallakarva@f555.n387.zl.fidonet.org (accessed February 18, 2007).

30. Ibid.

31. Ibid.

32. H J F Horstmanshoff, 1999. Ancient Medicine Between Hope and Fear: Medicament, Magic and Poison in the Roman Empire, *European Review* 7(1):37–51.

33. Ibid.

34. JH Trestrail, 2000. *Criminal Poisoning: Investigational Guide for Law Enforcement, Toxicologists, Forensic Scientists, and Attorneys,* Totowa, NJ: Humana Press.

35. H J F Horstmanshoff, 1999. Ancient Medicine Between Hope and Fear: Medicament, Magic and Poison in the Roman Empire, *European Review* 7(1):37–51.

36. Anil Aggrawal, 1997. The Poison Sleuths. Poisons, Antidotes, and Anecdotes. http://www.tripos.com/~Prof_Anil_Aggrawal/poiso001.html (accessed February 11, 2007).

37. H J F Horstmanshoff, 1999. Ancient Medicine Between Hope and Fear: Medicament, Magic and Poison in the Roman Empire, *European Review* 7(1):37–51.

38. CBWInfo, 2005. A Brief History of Chemical, Biological, and Radiological Weapons—Ancient Times to the 19th Century. http://www.cbwinfo.com/History/ancto19th.shtml (accessed February 17, 2007).

39. H J F Horstmanshoff, 1999. Ancient Medicine Between Hope and Fear: Medicament, Magic and Poison in the Roman Empire, *European Review* 7(1):37–51.

40. Ibid.

41. Smithsonian Magazine, 2004. Medicine from the Sea—From Slime to Sponges, Scientists Are Plumbing the Ocean's Depths for New Medications to Treat Cancer, Pain, and Other Ailments. http://www.smithsomianmagazine.com/issues/2004/may/medicine.htm (accessed February 20, 2007).

42. H J F Horstmanshoff, 1999. Ancient Medicine Between Hope and Fear: Medicament, Magic and Poison in the Roman Empire, *European Review* 7(1):37–51.

43. Hans Zinsser,1996. *Rats, Lice and History: A Chronicle of Disease, Plagues, and Pestilence*, New York: Black Dog & Leventhal Publishers, Inc.

44. Ibid.

45. H J F Horstmanshoff, 1999. Ancient Medicine Between Hope and Fear: Medicament, Magic and Poison in the Roman Empire, *European Review* 7(1):37–51.

46. Hans Zinsser,1996. *Rats, Lice and History: A Chronicle of Disease, Plagues, and Pestilence*, New York: Black Dog & Leventhal Publishers, Inc.

47. Ibid.

48. Gunnora Hallakarva, 1994. The Silent Weapon—Poisons and Antidotes in the Middle Ages. http://www.Gunnora.Hallakarva@f555.n387.zl.fidonet.org (accessed February 18, 2007).

49. John Kelly, 2005. *The Great Mortality, An Intimate History of the Black Death, the Most Devastating Plague of All Time*, New York: HarperCollins Publisher, Inc.

50. Jennifer Du, 2007. UCLA International Institute. Bioterrorism: How Has It Been Used? What Can It Do? How Prepared Are We? http://www.international.ucla.edu/article.asp?parentid=1352 (accessed February 12, 2007).

51. Ibid.

52. M. Cohen, 1989. *Health and the Rise of Civilization*, New Haven: Yale University Press.

53. CBWInfo, 2005. A Brief History of Chemical, Biological, and Radiological Weapons—Ancient Times to the 19th Century. http://www.cbwinfo.com/History/ancto19th.shtml (accessed February 17, 2007).

54. Anil Aggrawal, 1997. The Poison Sleuths. Poisons, Antidotes, and Anecdotes. http://www.tripos.com/~Prof_Anil_Aggrawal/poiso001.html (accessed February 11, 2007).

55. Portfolio MVM, 2007. Poisoning in the 16th, 17th, and 18th Century. http://www.portfolio.mvm.ed.ac.uk/studentwebs/session2/group12/16th.htm (accessed February 1, 2007).

56. Anil Aggrawal, 1997. The Poison Sleuths. Poisons, Antidotes, and Anecdotes. http://www.tripos.com/~Prof_Anil_Aggrawal/poiso001.html (accessed February 11, 2007).

57. Portfolio MVM, 2007. Poisoning in the 16th, 17th, and 18th Century. http://www.portfolio.mvm.ed.ac.uk/studentwebs/session2/group12/16th.htm (accessed February 1, 2007).

58. Anil Aggrawal,1997. The Poison Sleuths. Poisons, Antidotes, and Anecdotes. http://www.tripos.com/~Prof_Anil_Aggrawal/poiso001.html (accessed February 11, 2007).

59. Portfolio MVM, 2007. Poisons in the Renaissance. http://www.portfolio.mvm.ed.ac.uk/studentwebs/session2/group12/renaissance.html (accessed February 20, 2007).

60. Anil Aggrawal,1997. The Poison Sleuths. Poisons, Antidotes, and Anecdotes. http://www.tripos.com/~Prof_Anil_Aggrawal/poiso001.html (accessed February 11, 2007).

61. Ibid.

62. Portfolio MVM, 2007. Poisoning in the 16th, 17th, and 18th Century. http://www.portfolio.mvm.ed.ac.uk/studentwebs/session2/group12/16th.htm (accessed February 1, 2007).

63. Ibid.

64. Ibid.

65. Bio-Terry, 2007. History of Bioterrorism. A Chronological History of Bioterrorism and Biowarfare Throughout the Ages. http://www.bioterry.com/History BioTerr.html. (accessed February 16, 2007).

66. Ibid.

67. Ibid.

68. Ibid.

69. Portfolio MVM, 2007. Poisoning in the 16th, 17th, and 18th Century. http://www.portfolio.mvm.ed.ac.uk/studentwebs/session2/group12/16th.htm (accessed February 1, 2007).

70. Charles T. Gregg, 1985. *Plague: An Ancient Disease in the Twentieth Century,* Albuquerque: University of New Mexico Press.

71. 24-Hour Museum, 2004. Exhibitions. Rugeley Poisoner Returns to Stafford for New Exhibition. http://www.24hourmuseum.org.uk/exh_gfx_en/ART22617.html (accessed February 21, 2007).

72. Portfolio MVM, 2007. Madeleine Smith (1835–1928). http://www.portolio.mvm.ed.ac.uk/studentwebs/session2/group12/madeleine.html (accessed February 21, 2007).

73. Bio-Terry, 2007. History of Bioterrorism. A Chronological History of Bioterrorism and Biowarfare Throughout the Ages. http://www.bioterry.com/History BioTerr.html. (accessed February 16, 2007).

74. C. Loomis, 1991. *Weird and Tragic Shores: The story of Charles Francis Hall, Explorer,* Lincoln: Univ. Nebraska Press.

75. Ronald Bentley and Thomas G. Chasteen, 2001. Chem Educator. In the Classroom: Arsenic Curiosa and Humanity. http://www.chemeducator.org/sbibs/s0007002/spapers/720051rb.htm (accessed February 20, 2007).

76. J.H.H. Gaute and Robin Odell, 1996. *The New Murderer's Who's Who,* London: Harrap Books.

77. Portfolio MVM, 2007. Poisoning in the 20th Century. http://www.portfolio.mvm.ed.ac.uk/studentwebs/session2/group12/20th.htm (accessed February 22, 2007).

78. Bio-Terry, 2007. History of Bioterrorism. A Chronological History of Bioterrorism and Biowarfare Throughout the Ages. http://www.bioterry.com/HistoryBio Terr.html. (accessed February 16, 2007).

79. John M. Barry, 2004. *The Great Influenza: The Epic Story of the Greatest Plague in History,* New York, NY: Viking Penguin.

80. Geoff Simons, 1994. *Iraq: From Sumer to Saddam,* London: St. Martins Press.

81. Bio-Terry, 2007. History of Bioterrorism. A Chronological History of Bioterrorism and Biowarfare Throughout the Ages. http://www.bioterry.com/History BioTerr.html. (accessed February 16, 2007).

82. Ronald Bentley and Thomas G. Chasteen, 2001. Chem Educator. In the Classroom: Arsenic Curiosa and Humanity. http://www.chemeducator.org/sbibs/s 0007002/spapers/720051rb.htm (accessed February 20, 2007).

83. Bio-Terry, 2007. History of Bioterrorism. A Chronological History of Bioterrorism and Biowarfare Throughout the Ages. http://www.bioterry.com/HistoryBio Terr.html. (accessed February 16, 2007).

84. Ibid.

85. Ibid.

86. Ibid.

87. Portfolio MVM, 2007. Poisoning in the 20th Century. http://www.portfolio. mvm.ed.ac.uk/studentwebs/session2/group12/20th.htm (accessed February 22, 2007).

88. Ibid.

89. Ibid.

90. Eyewitness to History, 2007. The Forced Suicide of Field Marshall Rommel, 1944. http://www.eyewitnesstohistory.com/pfrommel.html (accessed February 21, 2007).

91. Jewish Virtual Library, 2007. The American-Israeli Cooperative Enterprise. Joseph Goebbels (1897–1945). http://www.jewishvirtuallibrary.org/jsource/ Holocaust/goebbels.html (accessed February 20, 2007).

92. Ibid.

93. Ibid.

94. Anil Aggrawal,1997. The Poison Sleuths. Poisons, Antidotes, and Anecdotes. http://www.tripos.com/~Prof_Anil_Aggrawal/poiso001.html (accessed February 11, 2007).

95. Ronald Bentley and Thomas G. Chasteen, 2001. Chem Educator. In the Classroom: Arsenic Curiosa and Humanity. http://www.chemeducator.org/sbibs/s 0007002/spapers/720051rb.htm (accessed February 20, 2007).

96. Anil Aggrawal,1997. The Poison Sleuths. Poisons, Antidotes, and Anecdotes. http://www.tripos.com/~Prof_Anil_Aggrawal/poiso001.html (accessed February 11, 2007).

97. A. Hodges, 1983. *Alan Turing: The Enigma,* New York: Simon & Shuster.

98. Ronald Bentley and Thomas G. Chasteen, 2001. Chem Educator. In the Classroom: Arsenic Curiosa and Humanity. http://www.chemeducator.org/sbibs/s 0007002/spapers/720051rb.htm (accessed February 20, 2007).

99. Bio-Terry, 2007. History of Bioterrorism. A Chronological History of Bioterrorism and Biowarfare Throughout the Ages. http://www.bioterry.com/History BioTerr.html. (accessed February 16, 2007).

100. Anil Aggrawal,1997. The Poison Sleuths. Poisons, Antidotes, and Anecdotes. http://www.tripos.com/~Prof_Anil_Aggrawal/poiso001.html (accessed February 11, 2007).

101. *TIME,*1978. TIME Archive: A Jury Sets Dr. X Free. http://www.time. com/time/printout/0,8816,948270,00.html (accessed February 16, 2007).

102. Bio-Terry, 2007. History of Bioterrorism. A Chronological History of Bioterrorism and Biowarfare Throughout the Ages. http://www.bioterry.com/HistoryBioTerr.html. (accessed February 16, 2007).

103. Ibid.

104. Portfolio MVM, 2007. Poisoning in the 20th Century. http://www.portfolio.mvm.ed.ac.uk/studentwebs/session2/group12/20th.htm (accessed February 22, 2007).

105. Ibid.

106. Bio-Terry, 2007. History of Bioterrorism. A Chronological History of Bioterrorism and Biowarfare Throughout the Ages. http://www.bioterry.com/HistoryBioTerr.html. (accessed February 16, 2007).

107. Ronald Bentley and Thomas G. Chasteen, 2001. Chem Educator. In the Classroom: Arsenic Curiosa and Humanity. http://www.chemeducator.org/sbibs/s0007002/spapers/720051rb.htm (accessed February 20, 2007).

108. Judith Mary Weightman, 1983. *Making Sense of the Jonestown Suicides*, New York: The Edwin Mellen Press.

109. Bio-Terry, 2007. History of Bioterrorism. A Chronological History of Bioterrorism and Biowarfare Throughout the Ages. http://www.bioterry.com/HistoryBioTerr.html. (accessed February 16, 2007).

110. Ibid.

111. ADL, 2005. Anti-Defamation League: Law Enforcement Agency Resource Network. Beyond Anthrax: Extremists and the Bioterrorism Threat. http://www.adl.org/learn/Anthrax/Earlier.asp?xpicked=2&item=4. (accessed February 22, 2007).

112. Barbara Mikkelson and David, 2006. Urban Legends Reference Pages. http://www.snopes.com/horrors/poison/tylenol.asp (accessed February 13, 2007).

113. Stuart C. Clarke, 2004. The Institute of Biomedical Science. Bioterrorism: past and current threats. http://www.ibms.org/index.cfm?method=science.general_science&subpage (accessed February 22, 2007).

114. Barbara Mikkelson and David, 2006. Urban Legends Reference Pages. http://www.snopes.com/horrors/poison/tylenol.asp (accessed February 13, 2007).

115. Stuart C. Clarke, 2004. The Institute of Biomedical Science. Bioterrorism: past and current threats. http://www.ibms.org/index.cfm?method=science.general_science&subpage (accessed February 22, 2007).

116. Paula Lampe, 2002. *The Mother Teresa Syndrome*, Holland: Nelissen.

117. CNN, 2006. Associated Press: Killer Nurse Gagged with Duct Tape at Sentencing. http://www.cnn.com/2006/LAW/03/10/killer.nurse.ap/index.html (accessed June 2, 2006).

118. Paula Lampe, 2002. *The Mother Teresa Syndrome*, Holland: Nelissen.

119. Barbara Mikkelson and David, 2006. Urban Legends Reference Pages. http://www.snopes.com/horrors/poison/tylenol.asp (accessed February 13, 2007).

120. Stuart C. Clarke, 2004. The Institute of Biomedical Science. Bioterrorism: past and current threats. http://www.ibms.org/index.cfm?method=science.general_science&subpage (accessed February 22, 2007).

121. Ibid.

122. Haruki Murakami, 1997. *Underground*. Translation by Alfred Birnbaum and Philip Gabriel. UK: Vintage Press.

123. Stuart C. Clarke, 2004. The Institute of Biomedical Science. Bioterrorism: Past and Current Threats. http://www.ibms.org/index.cfm?method=science.general_science&subpage (accessed February 22, 2007).

124. Bio-Terry, 2007. History of Bioterrorism. A Chronological History of Bioterrorism and Biowarfare Throughout the Ages. http://www.bioterry.com/HistoryBioTerr.html. (accessed February 16, 2007).

125. Stuart C. Clarke, 2004. The Institute of Biomedical Science. Bioterrorism: Past and Current Threats. http://www.ibms.org/index.cfm?method=science.general_science&subpage (accessed February 22, 2007).

126. Paula Lampe, 2002. *The Mother Teresa Syndrome*, Holland: Nelissen.

127. James B. Stewart, 1999. *Blind Eye—The Terrifying Story of a Doctor Who Got Away With Murder*, New York: Touchstone Books/Simon & Schuster.

128. Bio-Terry, 2007. History of Bioterrorism. A Chronological History of Bioterrorism and Biowarfare Throughout the Ages. http://www.bioterry.com/History BioTerr.html. (accessed February 16, 2007).

129. Ibid.

130. Ibid.

131. Ibid.

132. Mikaela Sitford, 2000. *Addicted to Murder*, UK: Virgin Publishing.

133. Paula Lampe, 2002. *The Mother Teresa Syndrome*, Holland: Nelissen.

134. Bio-Terry, 2007. History of Bioterrorism. A Chronological History of Bioterrorism and Biowarfare Throughout the Ages. http://www.bioterry.com/HistoryBioTerr.html. (accessed February 16, 2007).

135. Paula Lampe, 2002. *The Mother Teresa Syndrome*, Holland: Nelissen.

136. Bio-Terry, 2007. History of Bioterrorism. A Chronological History of Bioterrorism and Biowarfare Throughout the Ages. http://www.bioterry.com/HistoryBioTerr.html. (accessed February 16, 2007).

137. Paula Lampe, 2002. *The Mother Teresa Syndrome*, Holland: Nelissen.

138. Bio-Terry, 2007. History of Bioterrorism. A Chronological History of Bioterrorism and Biowarfare Throughout the Ages. http://www.bioterry.com/HistoryBioTerr.html. (accessed February 16, 2007).

139. Ibid.

140. Ibid.

141. BBC News, 2002. Russia Names Moscow Siege Gas. http://www.news.bbc.co.uk/1/hi/world/europe/2377563.stm (accessed February 15, 2007).

142. LookSmart, 2003. Christian Century: Arsenic Poisoning at a Maine Church. http://www.findarticle.com/p/articles/mi_m1058/is_10_120/ai_102140719/print (accessed February 13, 2007).

143. Paula Lampe, 2002. *The Mother Teresa Syndrome*, Holland: Nelissen.

144. Kaiser Papers, 2005. The Kaiser Papers. Reuters: Swiss Nurse is Sentenced for 22 Murders. http://www.kaiserpapers.org/swissnurse.html (accessed February 1, 2007).

145. *CBS News*, 2006. Katrina Doc Denies Mercy Killings. http://www.cbsnews.com/stories/2006/09/21/60minutes/printable2030603.shtml (accessed February 21, 2007).

146. CNN.com, 2006. Russian former spy dies. http://cnn.worldnews.printthis.clickability.com/pt/cpt?action=cpt&title=Russian+former(accessed February 22, 2007).

147. Karen Kaplan, Thomas H. Maugh II, 2007. LAtimes.com. Polonium-210's quiet trail of death. http://www.latimes.com/news/printedition/la-sci-polonium 1jan01,1,796078,print.story?ctr (accessed February 22, 2007).

Appendix B

1. Bill Holmes, 2007. Extensive Personal Interviews with Distributed Delivery Network's Principle Owner and Manager, from January through May 2007 (personal communication).

2. Pharmacy OneSource, 2007. Home page. High Performance Pharmacy Standardized. http://www.pharmacyonesource.com (accessed February 20, 2007).

3. *Drug Topics*, 2006. Will ATMs Replace You? http://www.drugtopics.com (accessed October 11, 2006).

4. Adam Dorin, November 2005. Drug ATMs: Will Physicians Go the Way of the Pharmacist? *San Diego County Medical Society PHYSICIAN.*

INDEX

About the Author

ADAM FREDERIC DORIN, M.D. is Medical Director at the SHARP Grossmont Plaza Surgery Center, and a Member-Shareholder of the Anesthesia Services Medical Group. He earned his premedical degree at the University of Maryland, completed his medical training at the University of Maryland School of Medicine, and completed his residency in anesthesiology and critical care medicine at Johns Hopkins University. Dr. Dorin also served as an officer in the U.S. Naval Reserve, where he attained the rank of lieutenant commander. He has been in private practice as an anesthesiologist and medical director for fifteen years. He has also been a volunteer surveyor of freestanding surgery centers across the nation.

For further information about *Jihad and American Medicine*, and an ongoing discussion about terrorism prevention in health care, see
http://www.JihadandAmericanMedicine.com,
http://www.PreventingMedicalTerrorism.com, or
http://www.AdamDorin.com.